This Book Will Make
You Feel Better

# This Book Will Make You Feel Better

SANDY BEACH

PENGUIN LIFE

AN IMPRINT OF

PENGUIN BOOKS

PENGUIN LIFE

UK | USA | Canada | Ireland | Australia
India | New Zealand | South Africa

Penguin Life is part of the Penguin Random House group of companies
whose addresses can be found at global.penguinrandomhouse.com.

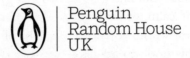

First published 2023
001

Copyright © Penguin Life, 2023

Illustrations by Josie Staveley-Taylor

The moral right of the copyright holder has been asserted

Set in 11.75/14pt Garamond MT Std
Typeset by Jouve (UK), Milton Keynes
Printed and bound in Great Britain by Clays Ltd, Elcograf S.p.A.

The authorized representative in the EEA is Penguin Random House Ireland,
Morrison Chambers, 32 Nassau Street, Dublin D02 YH68

A CIP catalogue record for this book is available from the British Library

ISBN: 978–0–241–65376–0

www.greenpenguin.co.uk

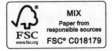

# How to Use This Book

Hello and welcome to the book designed to put a spring back in your step and bring a bit of sparkle to your day. Whether you're looking for a bit of inspiration, to boost your energy, to work that grey matter, find a bit of calm, or just simply a bit of distraction from the real world, you're in the right place. We've designed this book to act like your very own cheerleader, a safe space and source of creativity to turn to whenever you need it most.

Penguin Life is the home of wellbeing books, and this is our collection of the best mood-boosting tips and tricks all in one big, fun, messy list so that every time you pick it up you can flick through and land on something completely different. After all, variety is the spice of life, right?

We have included poems, jokes, exercises, games and crafting ideas and much, much more, all of which you can do with things lying around the house: whether that's some paper for making an origami swan, cushions and blankets for building a fort, or cards to learn a knock-out trick. There are also all sorts of comforting recipes to whip up when you fancy a treat, including the ultimate mug cake, fluffy pancakes and a to-die-for cheese toastie, which all use household ingredients.

You will find puzzles, doodling and colouring pages throughout the book, but don't feel limited to just drawing on those pages, let your creativity run free wherever you want to add your own personal touch! We would suggest using pencils to avoid ink running through to the other side of pages, but it's your book so go wild if you want. The only rules are, there are no rules.

We hope this book brings you some sunshine on the dark days, reminds you that you ARE enough, inspires you to try something new, to get outside, to dance like no one is watching, to let your emotions and creativity run free, to breathe a sigh of relief and feel just that bit better. You deserve it.

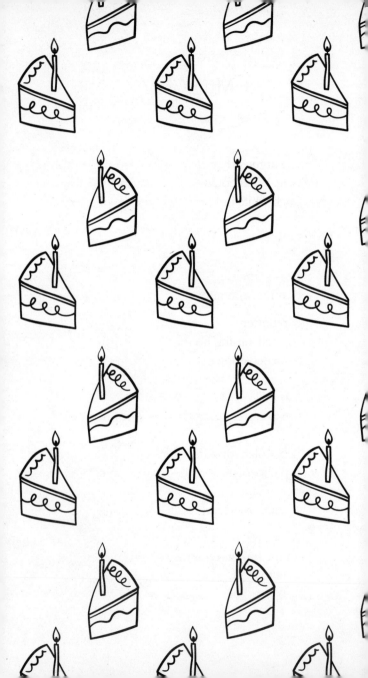

# Mug Cake

It could be argued that the most comforting thing *ever* is mug cake. What could be cosier than snuggling into a soft couch while holding a warm mug of cake?

Serves 1
Prep time – 5 minutes
Cooking time – 4 minutes

- 2 tbsp butter
- 3 tbsp self-raising flour
- 1 tbsp cocoa powder (optional)
- 1 egg
- 3 tbsp milk
- 2½ tbsp caster, granulated or soft brown sugar
- 25g chocolate or nuts, chopped
- 1 tbsp chocolate spread, caramel sauce, nut butter or jam
- Ice cream or cream, to serve (optional)

1. Take a large mug (about 300ml).
2. Add the butter, then microwave in 10-second bursts to melt.

3. Add the flour, cocoa powder (if using), egg, milk and sugar, and whisk until smooth.
4. Stir in the chocolate or nuts.
5. Dollop the chocolate spread, caramel sauce, nut butter or jam on top – it will sink into the batter to make a molten sauce.
6. Microwave for 2½–3 minutes on high until risen and firm.
7. Serve with ice cream or cream, to your taste.

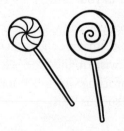

# Box-Breathing

The technique is as simple as its name: boxes have four equal sides, and thus the term 'box-breathing' was born. If you're feeling a little stressed, angry or overwhelmed, box-breathing can eliminate those feelings quickly. Box-breathing for one or two minutes can turn around negative emotions and help you when you feel triggered.

## *How to do it*

1. First, find a comfortable position, sitting or lying down, and relax your entire body.
2. Exhale fully for a count of four.
3. Hold and keep the lungs empty for a count of four.
4. Inhale for a count of four.
5. Hold the air in your lungs for a count of four.

While breathing, you can visualize a box. Then, with each breath or hold, imagine sliding across each side of the box in a clockwise or anti-clockwise direction. You can even say comforting words in your mind while you breathe and slide, such as 'I am calm' or 'I am here now'.

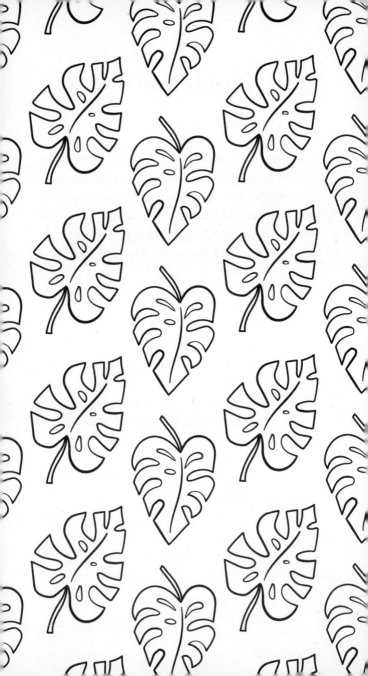

# Build a Fort

Too old to build a fort? Hell, no, you aren't. Making a blanket fort is great fun and a unique way to hang out at home – think of it as a staycation. Remember, your fort is *all* yours and can be used for listening to music, reading a book, writing your journal or (if they are lucky enough) hanging out with a friend or partner.

## *You will need the following*

- Two to four chairs
- Blankets or sheets to create the walls and roof
- A comfy blanket and cushions for the floor
- Stones or books to hold the roof in place
- Pegs for the doorway

## *How to make it*

1. Pick an area of your house to build your fort; you might need to rearrange the furniture to give you more space.

2. Place the chairs with the backs facing each other for the structure.
3. Drape blankets or sheets over the chairs to create the walls and roof.
4. Place the comfy blanket and cushions to make the floor.
5. To keep everything in place, you can position another blanket over the walls and ceiling.
6. Use heavy objects, like stones or books, to pin the covering to the floor.
7. Create a doorway by pinning back your sheets or blankets with pegs.

Enjoy being in your fort for as long as you can, and don't be surprised if you fall asleep in your cosy nest.

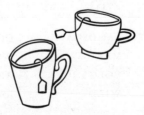

# Find These Words from Nature

| | | | | | |
|---|---|---|---|---|---|
| Y | P | N | G | P | X |
| W | O | D | A | E | M |
| M | C | R | G | S | E |
| F | E | W | N | L | N |
| L | A | R | H | Z | V |
| Q | N | A | N | B | I |
| I | R | I | V | E | R |
| L | O | N | Y | A | O |
| A | V | F | W | C | N |
| N | O | O | O | H | M |
| D | L | R | O | W | E |
| S | C | E | C | B | N |
| C | A | S | I | R | T |
| A | N | T | T | R | W |
| P | O | W | C | G | S |
| E | F | I | R | I | G |
| I | S | L | A | N | D |
| X | V | D | B | T | Y |

| | | |
|---|---|---|
| ENVIRONMENT | LANDSCAPE | OCEAN |
| ISLAND | MEADOW | WORLD |
| RIVER | VOLCANO | ARCTIC |
| BEACH | WILD | RAINFOREST |

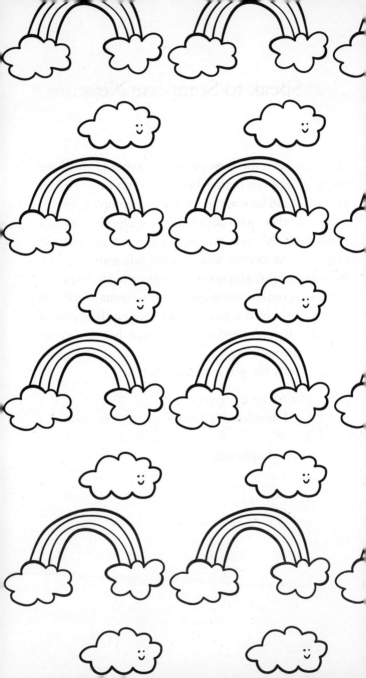

# Speak to Someone New

We've all been the 'new person' in school, work or a social group. No matter how outgoing or confident you are, it can be scary to walk into a group of friends and co-workers who already know each other. But it's not always the new person feeling out of place; it could be the person who doesn't talk much, maybe because they are shy, quiet and struggling to fit in.

So look out for anyone today who seems a little lost or unsure – why not go over and have a little chat with them? You don't need to be intrusive, but you might make someone's day.

Here are a few conversation starters:

- 'How's your day going?'
- 'Hey, I wondered if I could get your opinion on . . . ?'
- 'Where do you call home?'

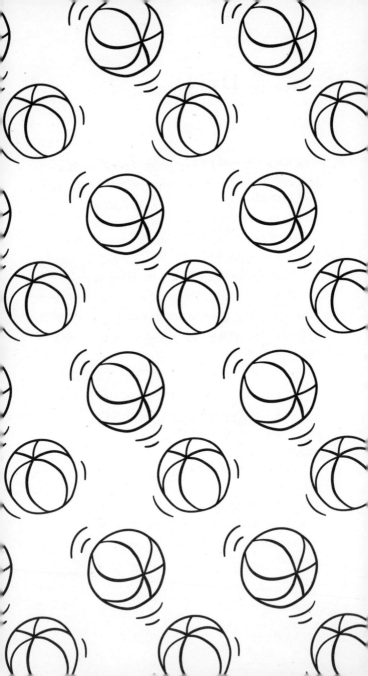

# Dad Jokes

We all love a good dad joke, don't we? No matter how corny or obvious they are, we all secretly love a pun and they provide a good old dose of wholesome fun to brighten up any day. Whether you're a dad yourself or have a soft spot for the classic one-liner, here are a few to add to your collection – just prepare yourself for a groan-worthy reaction next time you bring them out around the dinner table.

- I am getting so sick of millennials and their attitude. Always walking around like they rent the place.
- I asked a millennial yoga teacher to leave the room. He said: 'Nah a ma stay.'
- My wife told me to stop impersonating a flamingo. I had to put my foot down.
- When life gives you melons, you might be dyslexic.
- Russian dolls are so full of themselves.
- What's the difference between ignorance and apathy? I don't know and I don't care.

- I asked my date to meet me at the gym today. She didn't show up. That's when I knew we weren't going to work out.
- What did the number zero say to the number eight? Nice belt!
- I was wondering why the frisbee kept getting bigger, and then it hit me.

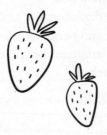

# Child's Pose

Child's Pose is also known as 'Balasana', which is derived from the Sanskrit word *bala*, which means 'childlike' and *asana*, meaning 'pose'. People say this pose brings out the stress-free inner child and reminds us of being in the womb. Child's Pose is simple and easy to do, even for people who have never tried yoga. It gently stretches your hip joints, lower back and upper shoulders and is the ideal posture in which to experience peace and stillness. Child's Pose is one of the most straightforward and intuitive yoga postures.

## *Benefits*

- Soothes tension and anxiety: placing the forehead on the floor is a wonderfully grounding experience.
- Improves the digestion and circulation.
- Relieves back and neck pain. As you reach forward, you lengthen the spine for a deep shoulder stretch and lower-back release.

Give it a try with the instructions on the next page!

## *How to do it*

1. Kneel down.
2. Lean forward, keeping your bottom on your heels, and gently place your forehead on the floor.
3. Place your arms loosely next to your legs, palms facing up, and enjoy an 'ahh' out-breath, breathing here slowly and mindfully.

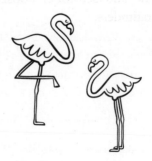

# Happy Memories

You know the scenario: you have a quiet moment, pull out your phone and, before you know it, you've been sucked into a vortex of social-media apps at the mercy of the algorithm. Unfortunately it happens to the best of us and doesn't always make us feel good. So here's a little hack to bypass a mindless scroll!

Spend five minutes making a photo folder in your phone named 'Happy Memories' and add all the images that make you smile. You can include photos of your 'happy people', beautiful places you have visited, delicious dinners you ate, your childhood home and perhaps screenshots of memorable conversations that made you smile. Then, whenever that quiet moment arrives, you simply bypass the apps and go straight into your 'Happy Memories' folder for a feel-good dopamine and serotonin boost and a sweet moment of gratitude.

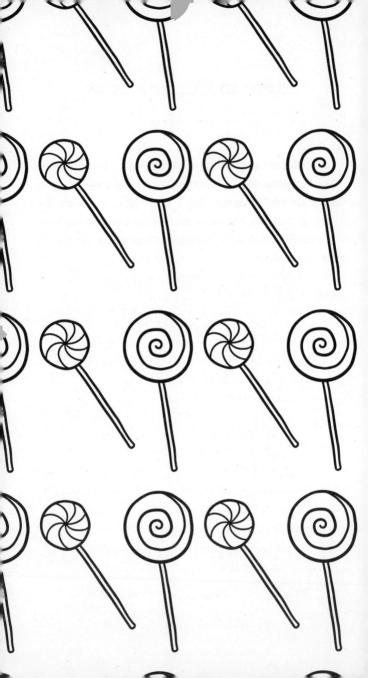

# Make an Origami Swan

Due to their long-standing symbolism of everlasting love, origami swans are frequently used as wedding and anniversary decorations. However, if you're not heading out to any nuptials soon, this swan decoration will look lovely hung up somewhere special in your home.

1. Start out with a square piece of paper and fold the bottom left-hand corner to the top right to create a diagonal fold. Now unfold it.
2. Next, fold the bottom edge and the right-hand side of the square into the diagonal centreline, so that it is kite shaped.
3. Turn the kite base around, so that the flaps are on the bottom side. Now fold the flaps back on themselves to meet the centreline, creating a narrower kite shape.
4. Next, fold the kite in half, bringing the bottom point of the kite to meet the top.
5. Then fold down the tip of the narrow point back on itself to create the beak. You can decide how big to make this but it should be shorter than the neck and body.

6. Next, fold the swan in half along the original fold down the middle of the kite shape so that it starts to stand up, and then gently pull the neck of the swan away from the body and the beak away from the neck, pinching it firmly until it stands up.
7. Behold, your beautiful swan!

*Voilà*, congratulations! Enjoy displaying your swan.

# Create a 'Go, Me' Folder

A 'Go, Me' folder is excellent for lifting your spirits at work if you're having a low-confidence day. Create a folder in your email, and save any emails that make you feel good. These might be compliments on your work, a 'yes' to a sale, the email that offered you the job or someone asking you to mentor them – anything you have received that makes you feel as if you're moving forward (which you always are). Stick it in your 'Go, Me' folder and have a little peek in there whenever you need a lift.

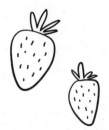

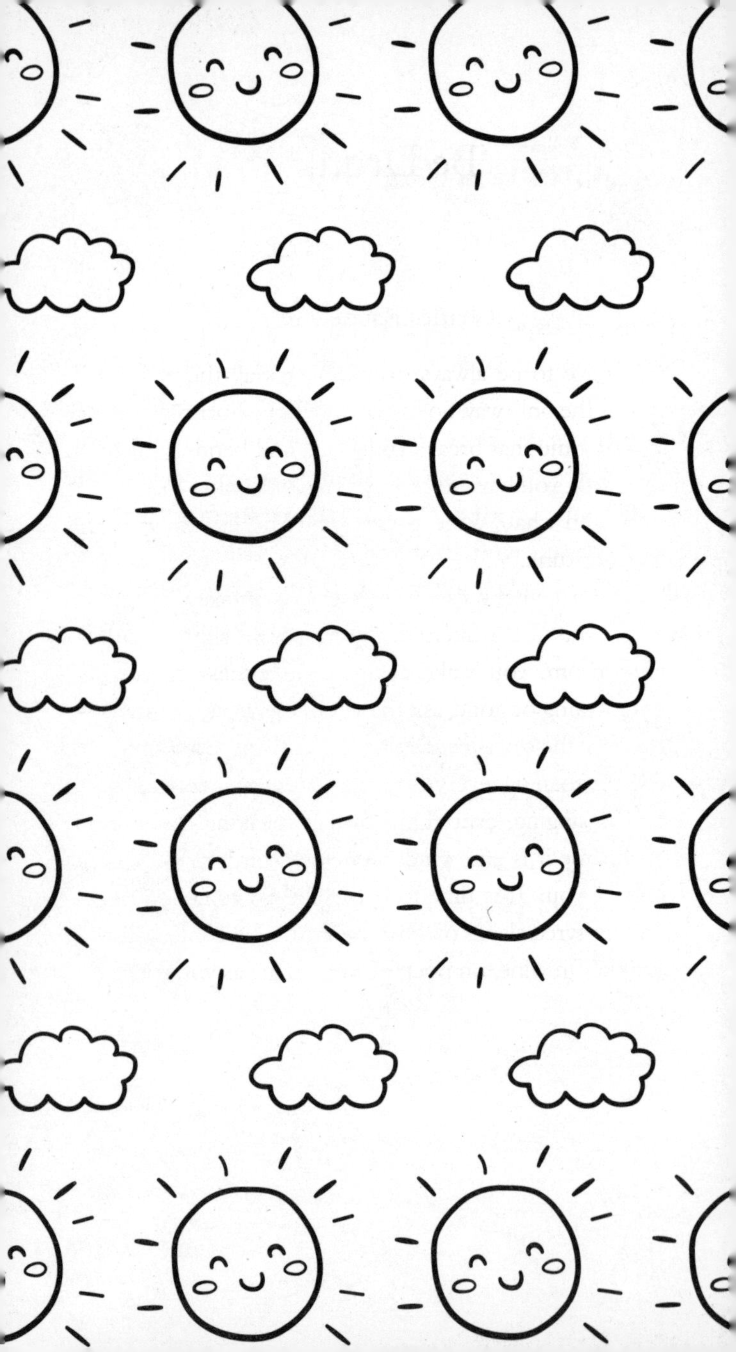

# 'Be Drunk'

## Charles Baudelaire

You have to be always drunk. That's all there is to it – it's the only way. So as not to feel the horrible burden of time that breaks your back and bends you to the earth, you have to be continually drunk.

But on what? Wine, poetry or virtue, as you wish. But be drunk.

And if sometimes, on the steps of a palace or the green grass of a ditch, in the mournful solitude of your room, you wake again, drunkenness already diminishing or gone, ask the wind, the wave, the star, the bird, the clock, everything that is flying, everything that is groaning, everything that is rolling, everything that is singing, everything that is speaking . . . ask what time it is and wind, wave, star, bird, clock will answer you: 'It is time to be drunk! So as not to be the martyred slaves of time, be drunk, be continually drunk! On wine, on poetry or on virtue as you wish.'

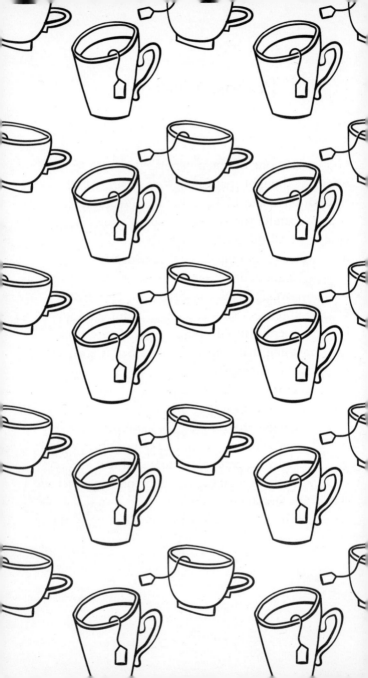

# Practise Gratitude

Gratitude is one of the most effective ways to reset negative thought patterns. The brain works by association – and by actively thinking about things you are grateful for, you will begin to remember and appreciate all the other things you are thankful for, thus switching your mindset and making you happier.

Practise gratitude by spending one or two minutes each day saying 'Thank you', in your head or out loud, for all the things that make you grateful. This could be your friends, health, home, pets, nature, and so on – anything that comes to mind. See it and say a huge thank-you with a smile.

Another way to practise gratitude is to write a gratitude journal. Each day write down three to five things that you are grateful for. Feel free to repeat the same ones, if they come up on multiple days. Then, after a month, read your gratitude entries and feel the serotonin whoosh through your body as you remember all the happy gratitude you've recorded – it's a great reminder that it ain't all so bad after all!

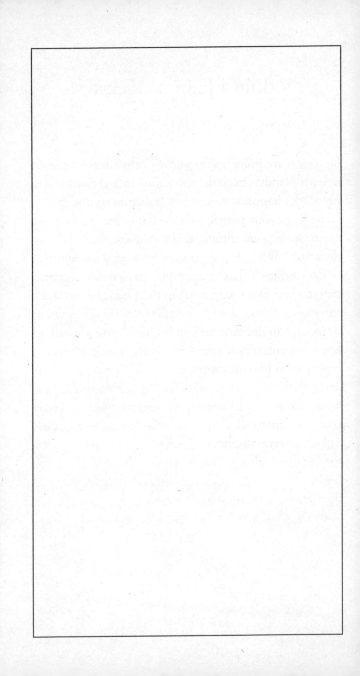

# Doodle a Happy Memory

Here you are going to doodle a happy memory. Have a pencil handy, check in with yourself and think back. Recall the happiest memory that comes to mind.

Pick up your pencil with that specific memory in mind. Ask your intuition: what does this memory look like? What shape or size is it? Is it an abstract shape or does it have features, like a person or an animal would? Does this memory have jagged, scratchy or smooth lines?

Just begin drawing and allow your hand to express the emotion. Then when you have finished, take a moment to look at the drawing and accept it as part of you. This offers your subconscious validation, which gives you an opportunity to see how you view your own memories.

Happy reminiscing!

# The Perfect Bath

You're about to learn what you might already have suspected to be true: there *is* such a thing as the perfect bath. While philosophers have debated the formula for millennia (don't fact-check us!), the most recent agreement is that there *is* a perfect bath. Now you know that a bath doesn't have to be *just* a bath, here is a recipe that will give you a better chance of achieving that dreamy experience.

1. Make sure you have drawn a line under all the tasks in your day and that you can go to bed immediately, post-bath.

2. Temperature is key! The hot water should be running, but you should also have the cold water running slightly, so that the water isn't scalding when you get in. Of course, water temperature is a matter a preference, so use your wrist (not your hand) to determine the perfect warmth. If you want bubbles, you should pour them in at the beginning to allow them to build while the bath fills.

3. While the water is running, you can calmly collect any of the following items: candles, bath salts, bath oil, a good book, music,

snacks, a beverage of your choice or a lavender diffuser.

4. Before the bath is full and you've taken off all your clothes, check that the water is at a temperature you can dip a foot into without yelping. Adjust accordingly, if necessary.

5. Light the candles, turn on the diffuser, set up the speaker with your ideal playlist and then pour in the bath salts and oil.

6. Sink into your bespoke water-sanctuary and breathe in the well-earned peace.

# The Great Outdoors

You've decided to go for a walk: wonderful! Shoes and coat on, you step out, but suddenly you get so wrapped up in your thoughts and inner dialogue that you forget to notice the elements and the magnificence of nature around you.

Even if you live in a city, nature finds a way – it's everywhere! If you pay attention, just for a short time, you can remind yourself how glorious the planet is. Here are some elements of nature to look out for when you're putting one leg in front of the other:

- What colour is the sky? Not just blue or grey: what sort of shade?
- What sort of birds can you see? Are there any perching in bushes?
- Are there any flowers you can see growing wild or in gardens, on windowsills?
- What can you smell? Log-burners, cut grass or rain on the pavement?
- Are there any dogs being walked? Are they excited to be outside too?

# Let It Out

'Stiff upper lip', 'stoicism', 'keep calm and carry on' – sound familiar? These concepts are great until the feelings you have inside begin to suffocate you. So here is your reminder that sometimes it's okay to let it all out. Crying and emotion are aspects of life for which you never need to apologize.

So if you feel overwhelmed by your emotions, take a moment to be present and think about what is bothering you. Let that take over your feelings, and allow your anger/frustration/sadness to come out. Scream into a cushion, rip apart a cardboard box or cry on the floor. Allow the feelings to come, and then witness them leave. Say, 'Thank you for the lesson'. Acknowledging your emotions makes it easier to release them, and uniting gratitude with discomfort can help you to move forward.

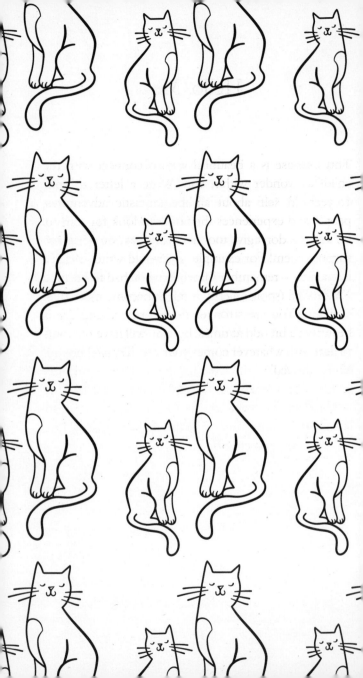

# Hello, Me

This exercise is a beautiful way to connect with the childlike wonder within you. Write a letter to your 10-year-old self about all the fantastic adventures, people and experiences they have to look forward to. Of course, don't give too much away, as you want it to surprise them! For example, you could write, 'Believe in yourself – remember that dream you had to become XYZ? Well (spoiler alert!), it might become more than a dream. You are stronger than you feel, and life is beautiful; a bit odd at times, but you will have the tools to deal with whatever comes your way. Try *all* the food. You are loved!'

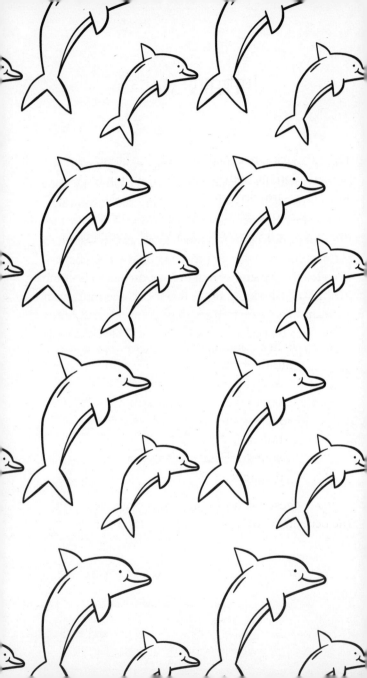

# Jumping Jacks

Jumping Jacks are a fun way to get the blood pumping and wake up the body when you're feeling fatigued or low. They are also great for cardiovascular health, increasing bone density and boosting metabolism, so give it a go – it's your choice if you wait until you're in private!

## *How to do them*

1. Begin in a standing position, with your hands on your thighs and your knees slightly bent.
2. While keeping the knees bent, your arms come out to the side, then above the head, and your legs should jump out wider than your shoulders.
3. Close your arms and your legs back to your sides, then repeat.

We suggest you do 50 of these a day to truly enjoy the benefits of your new Jumping Jack lifestyle.

# Donate

Many countries across the world have been affected by the economic crisis following the pandemic and the war in Ukraine so the need for food banks has increased dramatically. For the first time the number of people in need will exceed the number of people able to provide aid, highlighting the critical necessity for individuals to contribute to their local food banks.

It's simple to help those in need while grocery-shopping, as most supermarkets feature collection boxes for local food banks. Monetary donations are gratefully accepted, if you cannot collect and contribute goods.

Donations need not be astronomical. You can make a massive difference in helping those in need, even if it's just by purchasing a few additional items during your regular shopping trip and putting them in the collection boxes, or contributing money to a food bank.

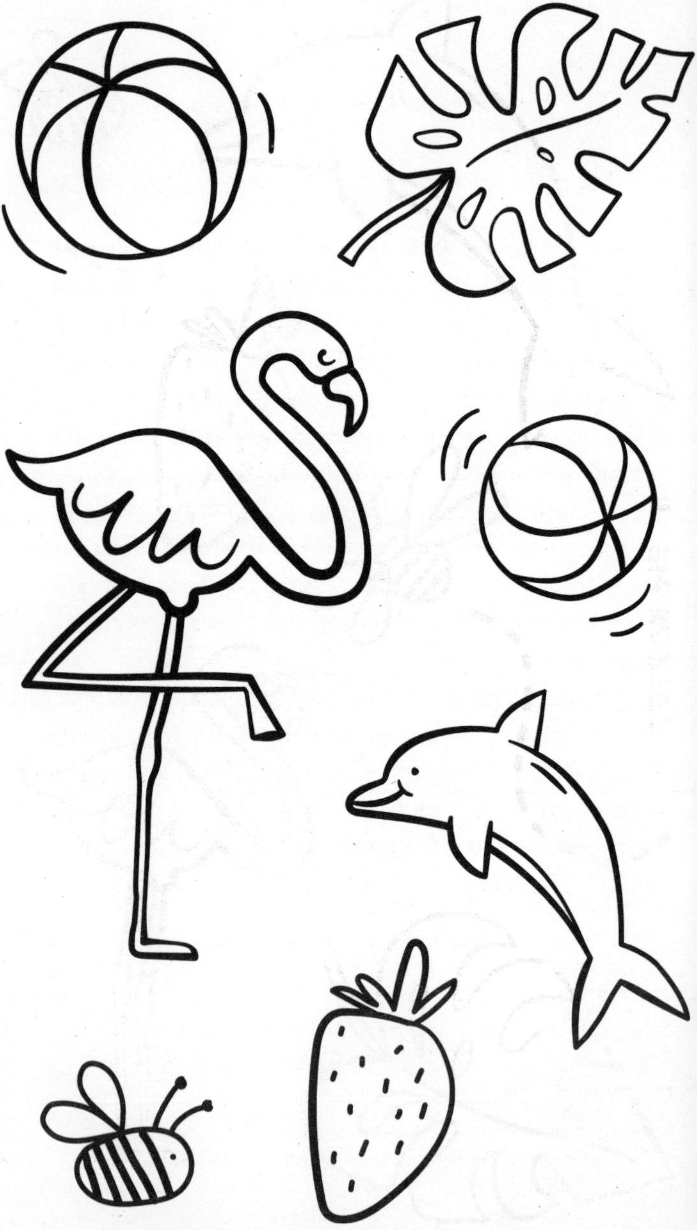

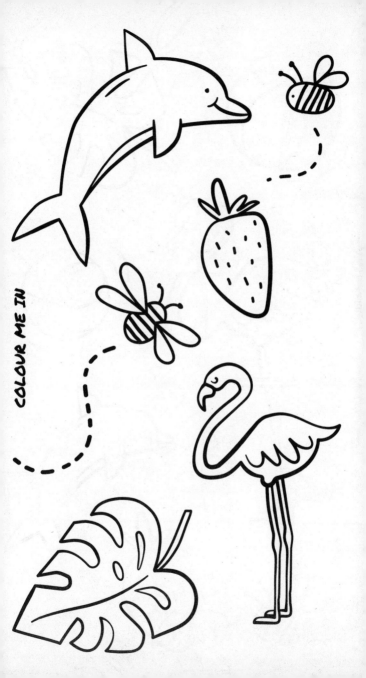

COLOUR ME IN

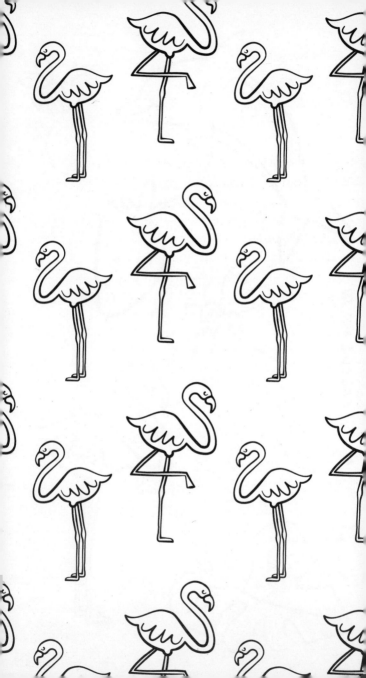

# Feel-Good News: Lost species returned in 2022

It was reported that many creatures grew exponentially in numbers in late 2022, proving that extinction may not be the inevitability it was once thought.

Most are the subject of reintroduction programmes, including the bison, which are now wandering the fields of the UK for the first time in several thousand years. Beavers and pelicans have also made a remarkable comeback.

Rhinos have returned to Mozambique, and there have been reports of a revival of fin whales and tigers.

These re-emerging species give us hope that one day we could see reintroductions of other animals on a much larger scale.

(positive.news)

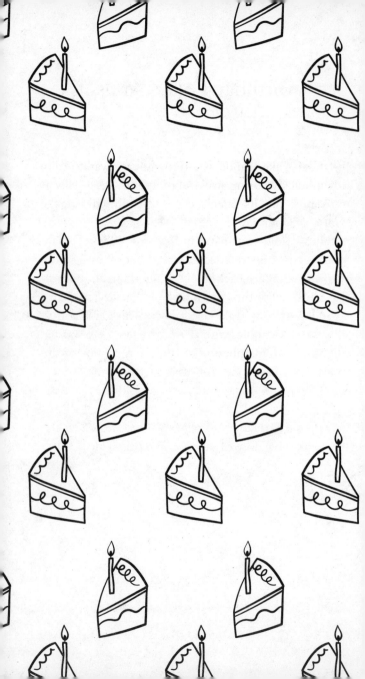

# Birthday-Cake Hands

'Birthday-Cake Hands' is a fun and easy way to calm down quickly during stressful moments. It's as silly as it sounds, but its effects can positively change the course of your day.

Simply hold your hand in front of your face with your fingers outstretched and palm facing away from you, and visualize each finger as a colourful, lit birthday candle, with the flames flickering gently, ready for you to blow out. Take a big breath in and begin to blow out the candles with all the force you can muster, one by one, remembering to take a large, juicy breath in between each one. As each candle is blown out, bend the finger down until you have blown out all the candles.

Afterwards, take a moment to notice how you feel (probably a big dose of 'ahh'), and repeat if necessary.

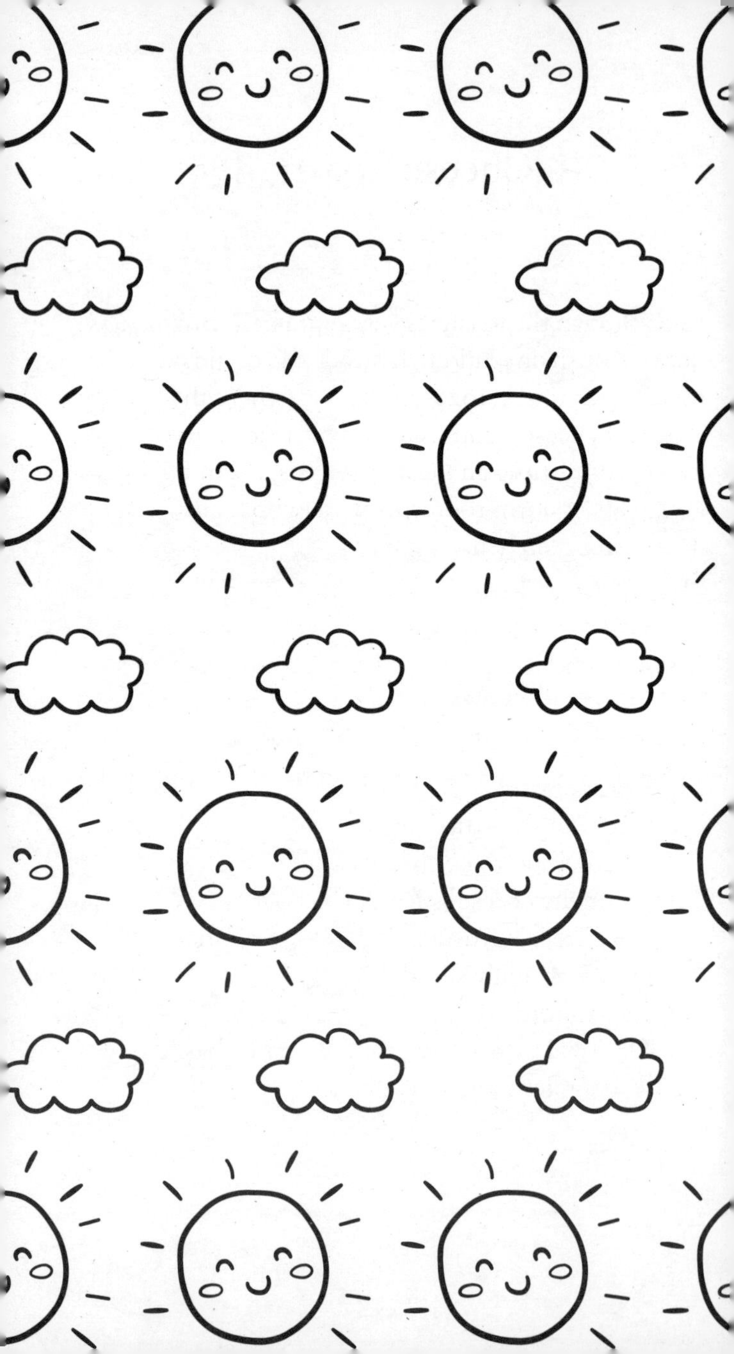

# Cheese Toastie

Even though the toastie is very popular in Britain, it is not a British invention. Instead the origins can be traced back to the 1920s in the US (where they call it a grilled-cheese sandwich – which adds up!). The warm, comforting and tasty toastie is a firm favourite in university dorm rooms, at workpeople's desks and, now, in your kitchen.

Serves 1
Prep time – 5 minutes
Cooking time – 5 minutes

- 2 slices bread
- Butter or mayo, to spread
- Chutney, pesto or chilli jam
- 50g melty cheese (such as Cheddar, mozzarella, Gruyère, Red Leicester, Brie), grated or thinly sliced
- 2 slices tomato
- Optional extras: ham, pastrami, torn basil leaves, sliced gherkin

1. Spread both slices of bread with butter or mayo.
2. Turn the bread so that the buttered sides are facing down.
3. Spread a little chutney, pesto or chilli jam on one slice, then top with the cheese and slices of tomato.
4. Close the sandwich with the second slice, so that the buttered side is facing up.
5. Heat a non-stick pan over a medium heat and add the sandwich.
6. Press down on it with a spatula for 2–3 minutes until the toast is golden, then flip and toast for another 1–2 minutes until the cheese has melted.
7. Devour!

# Dance Like an Idiot

For a quick boost of feel-good endorphins and sero-tonin, there is nothing like dancing like an idiot. This exercise can be accomplished at any time of day and in any location. Of course, try not to get fired from your job, but otherwise you do *you*!

We're sure you've danced like an idiot before, but if you've aged a year and have forgotten, here are the rules:

1. Throw on a song that you love.
2. Turn up the volume and let it all out.
3. Dancing like an idiot works best if you engage all the limbs *and* the head. For extra fun, jumping around really packs a punch.
4. To truly top off this miraculously happy activity, sing along loudly and grin like a Cheshire cat for the entirety of the song.
5. Job done! Rinse and repeat.

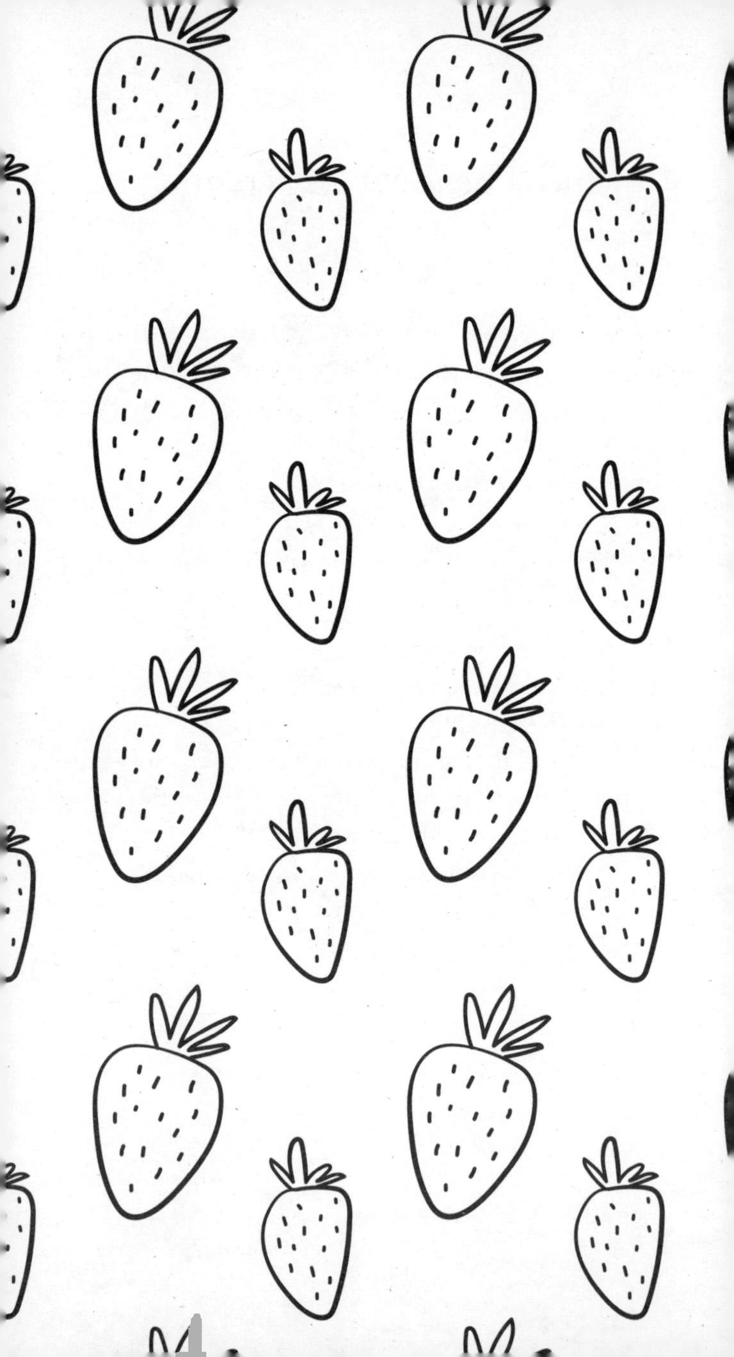

# Find These Sweet Treats

| | | | | | |
|---|---|---|---|---|---|
| L | T | N | X | W | E |
| P | O | K | R | L | R |
| N | L | L | F | K | V |
| Q | T | I | L | I | R |
| A | R | G | F | Y | T |
| T | B | S | B | Y | H |
| G | I | C | I | N | G |
| O | S | Z | A | Y | I |
| B | C | W | E | K | L |
| S | U | U | B | B | E |
| T | I | X | O | P | D |
| O | T | E | N | E | H |
| P | I | C | B | I | S |
| P | E | L | O | N | I |
| E | N | T | N | W | K |
| R | O | N | A | O | R |
| N | C | R | Q | R | U |
| I | S | I | P | B | T |

TART            SCONE           PIE
ICING           LOLLY           TRIFLE
BISCUIT         CAKE            GOBSTOPPER
BROWNIE         BONBON          TURKISH DELIGHT

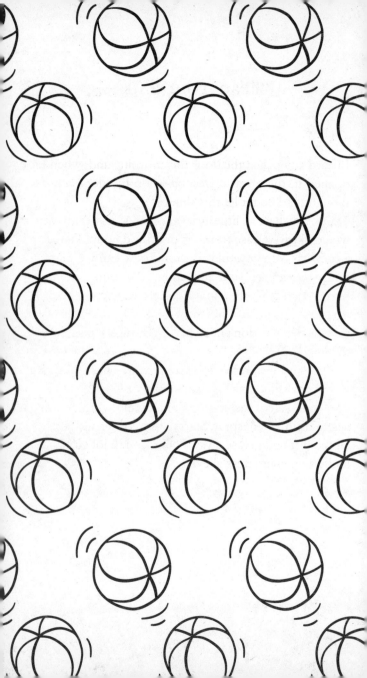

# Clean Your Sink

I heard a knock at the door this morning and, when I opened it, there was a washbasin on the doorstep. I thought, 'I'd better let this sink in.'

Do you have a little grievance or stress that you would like to release from the mind and body? Here is a trick Mr Miyagi would be proud of: clean your sink until you can see your reflection. Of course, if you have a matt sink, the same rules apply; you are going for 'straight out of the showroom' clean! The best thing is that you don't need harsh chemicals to achieve the goal.

Avoid using abrasive tools, like a wire brush, as this will scratch the sink, so use cloths instead. You will need hot water, washing-up liquid, white vinegar and a light disinfectant spray. Start in one corner and scrub all the dirt and grease away. Focus on the job at hand and watch your stress alleviate.

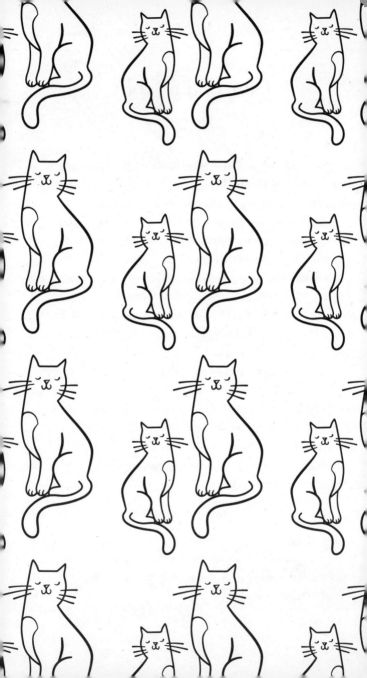

# Hello, Old Friend

Many of us fall into the trap of spending too much time worrying about the future, waiting for our next trip away or working towards our next promotion, but if we don't make enough time for our friendships, they can sometimes fall by the wayside. If there is someone in your life that you've lost touch with or really miss, why not write them a letter?

First, it's paramount that you take a quiet moment to remember all the things you admired and loved about the recipient. Then keep those qualities in mind as you write your letter.

You could write about joint adventures and remind them of an in-joke you shared. While recalling events and writing to this person, you might be surprised to refind a part of yourself – a unique piece of you that you thought you'd lost.

Remember, you don't *have* to send the letter; it's primarily about the process. However, if you're feeling good about it, stick a stamp on it or hit send and make someone's day!

Try smiling as you compose your letter – it can improve your writing tone and make you sound much friendlier, happier and more confident. Enjoy, and good luck, old friend.

# Learn a Dance Routine

Since the advent of TikTok, learning a dance routine has become part and parcel of teenage life, but whether that's you or not, hopefully 'The Macarena', 'YMCA', 'Saturday Night' and 'Candy' might ring a bell.

If you don't know or can't remember the dances to those songs, stick them on YouTube and watch a tutorial. Learning anything is always good for the neural pathways, especially when it incorporates coordination, patterns and rhythm. Why not leave your comfort zone and learn a song from a different generation or culture? You might discover a new passion for a musical genre or dance style.

If you're wondering what to do with your new dance routine, it's simple. Let's dance like it's 1999, blast our chosen song all over the house (or jukebox) and do it for the kicks.

# Doodle How You're Feeling

Here you are simply going to express how you're feeling through the art of doodling. Have a pencil handy, close your eyes and check in with yourself. How are you feeling? Is there an emotion that comes to mind? Are you happy, sad, scared, excited, jealous, in love or inspired? The first thing that comes to mind is probably the emotion you are feeling the most right now.

Pick up your pencil with that specific emotion in mind. Ask your intuition: what does this emotion look like? What shape or size is it? Is it an abstract shape or does it have features, like a person or an animal would? Does this emotion have jagged, scratchy or smooth lines?

Just begin drawing and allow your hand to express the emotion. Then when you have finished, take a moment to look at the drawing and accept it as part of you. This offers your subconscious validation, which can in turn allow you to release or integrate the emotion – whatever feels right for you.

Be true to yourself and enjoy the process.

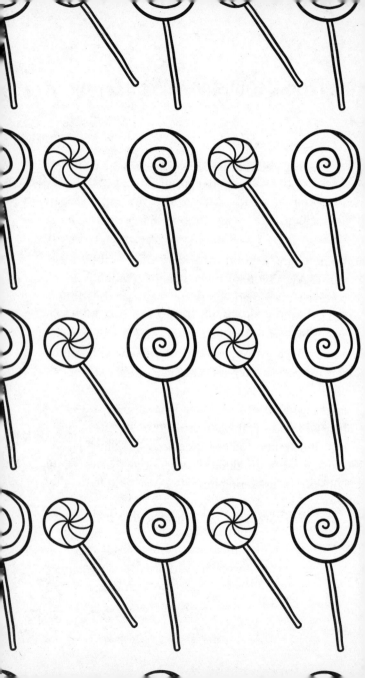

# Sign Up to Volunteer

The smallest act of kindness is worth more than the
grandest intention.

– Oscar Wilde

Volunteering is good for your mental health because
it gives you a sense of purpose and community, boosts
your self-esteem and gives you a chance to learn new
skills. Volunteering might make you think of flying
around the world to help in disaster zones, which is
admirable; however, you can also volunteer and be of
service on a smaller scale and still make a huge difference. There are many ways to give back, so it's best to
list the things you are passionate about, as this will
help you find suitable volunteer projects. Next, decide
how much time you could dedicate to volunteering.

Here are some different categories that you could
consider volunteering in:

- Environmental work – conservation, etc.
- Animals – animal rescue, etc.
- Social work – mentoring, etc.
- Healthcare – working with the elderly, etc.
- Sports and leisure – working with kids, etc.

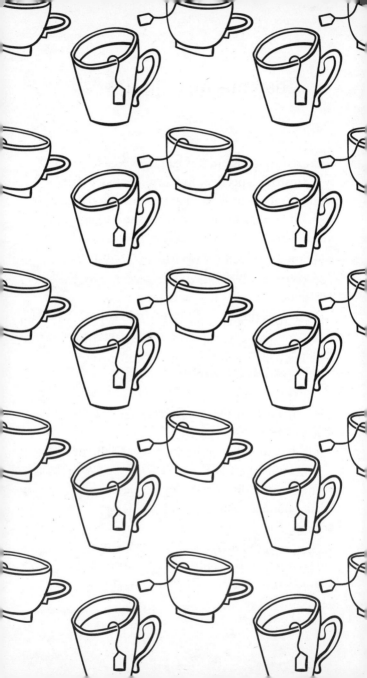

# Inspirational Quotes

Wise words from wise minds can help you see things from a fresh perspective and inspire you to think about things differently. Sometimes hearing the right words is all it takes to guide you forward, to give you the confidence you need to take your next steps, to navigate the world with awareness and, ultimately, to improve your mindset. Here are a few incredible quotes to lift you:

- 'Keep away from people who try to belittle your ambitions. Small people always do that, but the really great make you feel that you, too, can become great' – Mark Twain
- 'Just one small positive thought in the morning can change your whole day' – Dalai Lama
- 'It is never too late to be what you might have been' – George Eliot
- 'The greatest discovery of my generation is that a human being can alter his life by altering his attitudes' – William James
- 'You cannot plough a field by turning it over in your mind. To begin, begin' – Gordon B. Hinckley

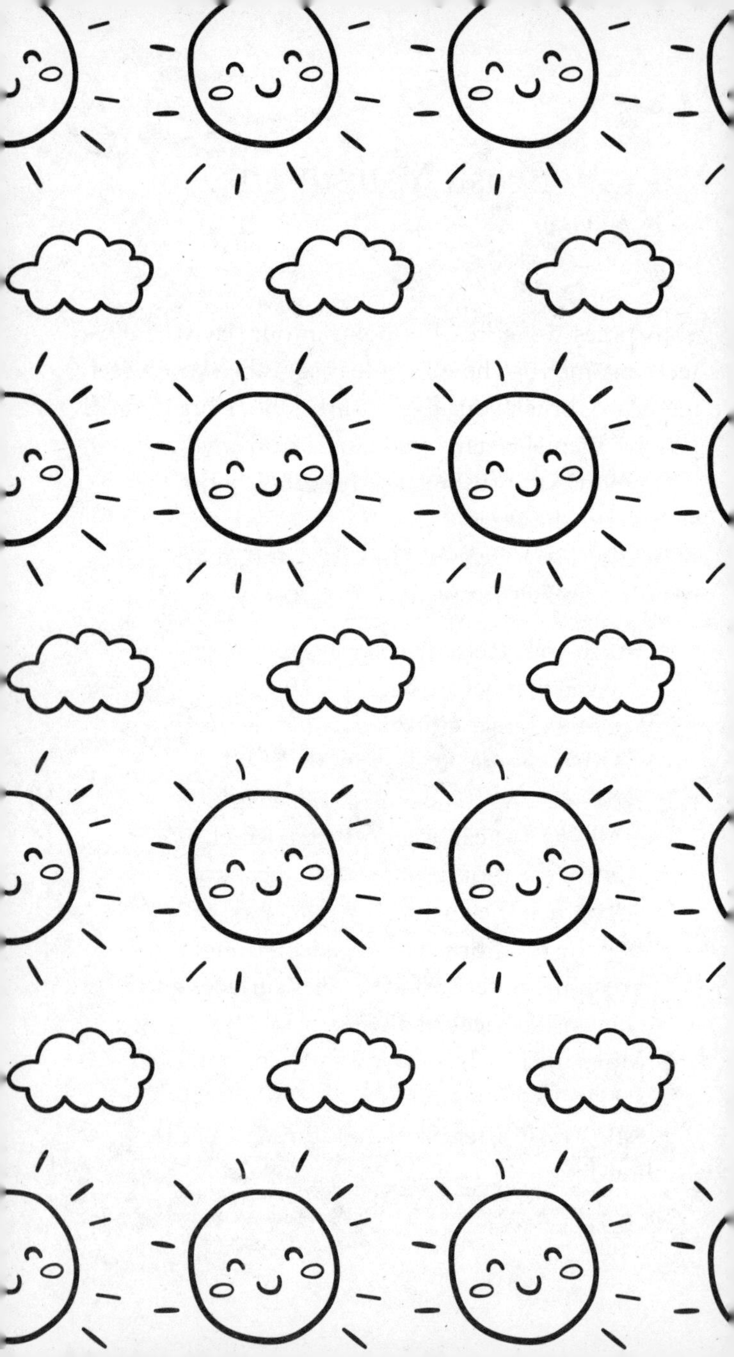

# Brush Your Teeth

Sometimes we all reach a point in our day where we feel a bit 'meh', so here's a little trick. When you're feeling down, brush your teeth, to trick your brain into a positive mental restart, ready to take on anything!

Speaking of brushing teeth, we all know that we should brush at least twice a day, but are you doing it correctly? Here are a few tips to ensure that the time spent brushing your teeth is productive.

- Brush your teeth twice a day, once during the day and just before bed.
- Flossing: unlike brushing, you only need to do this once daily, ideally at night.
- Don't brush after eating or drinking anything acidic, as this can wear off the enamel.
- Always use toothpaste with fluoride to strengthen the enamel.
- Use the toothbrush at a 45-degree angle and brush the outer surfaces, inner surfaces and chewing surfaces of the teeth.
- Move the brush back and forth in tooth-wide strokes.
- Don't rinse after brushing; spit out the excess toothpaste.

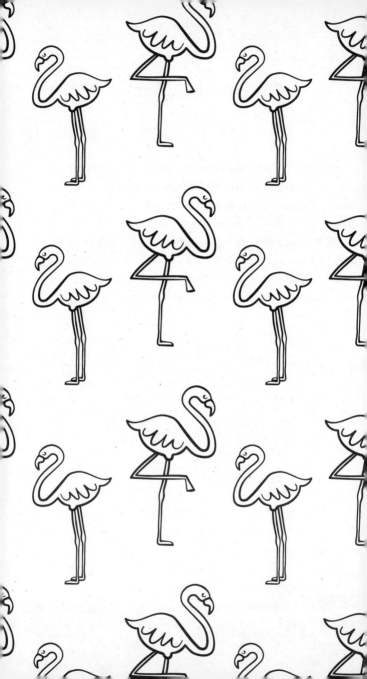

# Joke: Wild Cargo

A man was driving down the road when a policeman stopped him and asked if he could look in the back of the man's van. Upon seeing his cargo, he asked, 'Why do you have these penguins in your van?'

'Well, these are my penguins, you see. I own them,' the man replied.

'Well, you can't just be driving around dilly-dallying with penguins. You need to take them to the zoo!' the policeman said.

The man in the van agreed, and they parted ways.

Two days later the policeman saw the same man in the same van driving down the road. Suspicious, he pulled him over and saw that the penguins were still in the van, and they were all wearing sunglasses this time.

'Sir, I told you that you needed to take these penguins to the zoo!' the policeman said.

'I did,' the man replied, 'and today I'm taking them to the beach.'

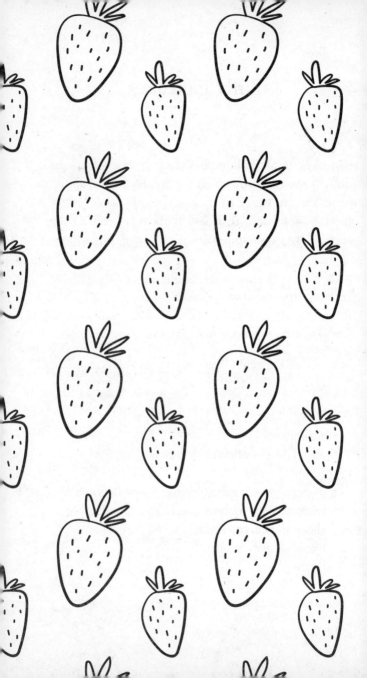

# Fluffy Pancakes

Pancakes in the traditional American style – thick and fluffy – are a delicious treat for Sunday brunch. Fluffy pancakes are easier to make than they look, so you should cook more than you think you need, as they are likely to get snapped up quickly by guests.

Serves 2 (makes 6 pancakes)
Prep time – 5 minutes
Cooking time – 10–15 minutes

- 125g self-raising flour
- 1 tsp baking powder
- 1 tbsp sugar
- 1 egg
- 100ml milk
- Vegetable, sunflower or rapeseed oil for frying
- Topping ideas: salted butter, crispy bacon and maple syrup, yoghurt and berries, fried apple slices and caramel sauce, sliced banana and hot-chocolate sauce

1. Mix the flour, baking powder and sugar together in a jug.
2. Beat in the egg, then slowly whisk in the milk until the batter is thick and smooth. (Alternatively, blend together in one go using a stick-blender.)
3. Heat a little oil in a flat non-stick pan.
4. Cook the pancakes in batches of two or three, depending on the size of the pan.
5. Spoon in 3 tbsp of mixture per pancake and cook on a low–medium heat for 2–3 minutes, until the pancakes have set around the edge and bubbles are starting to form on the surface.
6. Flip the pancakes and cook for another 1–2 minutes until golden and firm.
7. Divide between two plates and serve with your favourite topping.

# The Salutation Pose

This is one of the most popular 'power poses', which instantly activates your potential and gives you an express route to becoming more grounded, present and powerful.

## *How to do it*

1. Start by standing with your feet together and firmly planted on the floor.
2. Then, drawing your navel towards your spine, reach your arms in front of you with your palms facing upwards.
3. This is one of the most expansive poses you can strike; after maintaining it for a minute, you can't help but experience a surge of vitality, strength and confidence.

And remember: you *deserve* to feel this way!

# Feel-Good News: 95-year-old Grammy winner

At 95 years old, Angela Álvarez is the oldest person to be nominated and win 'best new artist' at the Latin Grammys.

Álvarez told Spanish news agency EFE that she began writing songs in 1942 in Cuba, but it took her 80 years to release her first album, encouraged by her grandson.

On her win, Angela said, 'It's indescribable. What I feel is such a wonderful and beautiful thing, and I can't find the words to express what I really feel. I feel very happy and content and very proud of what has happened in my life.'

Angela is a reminder to us all that it's never too late to pursue your ambitions and dreams.

(euronews.com)

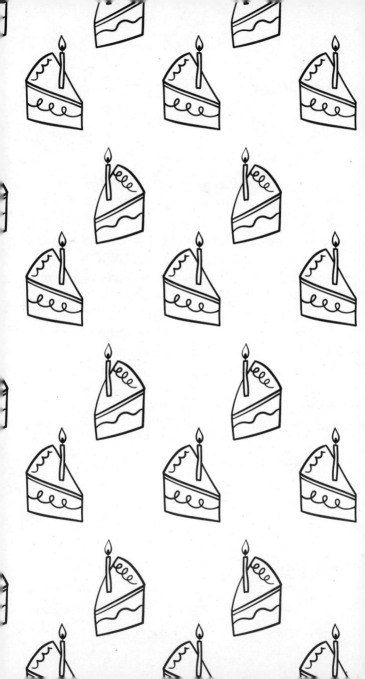

# The Power-of-Music Playlist

Make a personalized playlist on Spotify that is guaranteed to get your head bobbing and the serotonin surging. If you're like 90 per cent of the population and you can't resist getting cheery when you hear 'Good Vibrations' by the Beach Boys or 'Good as Hell' by Lizzo, then 'The Power-of-Music Playlist' is going to work for you. Putting together your happy playlist can take a little time (we suggest spending five minutes here and there, when you would otherwise be scrolling through your socials), but we guarantee you will enjoy the process!

Here are some artists to get you started:

- Lizzo
- The Beach Boys
- Marvin Gaye
- Queen
- James Brown
- Kool & the Gang
- Paul Simon
- George Michael
- Stevie Wonder
- Diana Ross

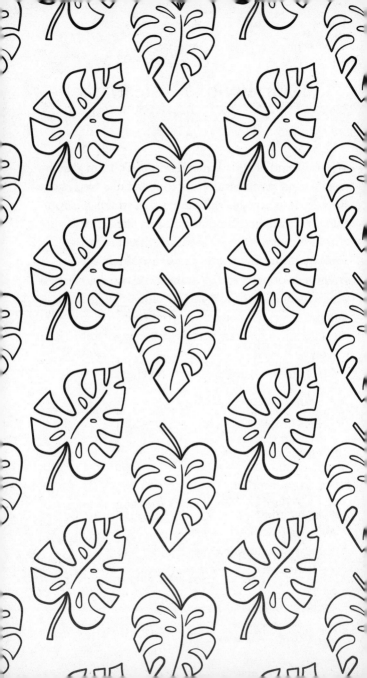

# Four, Four, Six Breathing Technique

If your mind is whirring and you can't seem to calm down, then pay attention to your breath. No matter how anxious you are, remember that worry can't hurt you – you will get through this, just like you have got through every other setback in your life. Simply follow the four, four, six breathing pattern and your body will soon get the message to relax.

1. Take a deep breath in through your nose for a count of four.
2. Hold for four breaths.
3. Exhale fully through your mouth for six counts.

Allow these breaths to be noisy and deep. Pay attention to the sound when you breathe in through your nose, how still and calm you feel when you hold your breath, and the sound when you breathe out through your mouth.

Repeat until you feel your heartbeat getting slower.

# Make an Origami Heart

Origami paper hearts are usually presented as a wedding gift, wishing the couple a thousand years of happiness and success, but this is also a fun new skill to learn and a relaxing way to spend a few minutes.

1. Begin with a square piece of paper. You can easily create this from an A4 sheet by folding the top left or right corner to the opposing sides to create a triangle of folded paper with a rectangle of unfolded paper at the bottom. Fold this rectangle backwards to create a neat line at the bottom of the triangle and then cut along that line and unfold the triangle to create a perfect square.
2. Start with points of the square at the top and bottom and fold the paper in half by folding the bottom corner to the top corner and then unfold till flat.
3. Repeat by folding the left corner to the right and then unfold
4. Fold the top corner to the centre crease (creating a diamond shape).
5. Fold the bottom corner to the middle of the top edge.

6. Fold the bottom right-hand corner upwards so that it lines up with the same middle top edge, then repeat on the left side.

7. This should now resemble a heart but to perfect your shape, flip it over and fold back the top and side corners to create four small triangles at the back and give your heart straight sides.

8. Flip the paper over – and take a big, happy look at your heart!

# Make Your Own Face Mask

If you feel like a pamper-day, but don't wish to go out and spend a small fortune, you can easily make a refreshing face mask from items in your home. It's simple.

## *Face Mask with two ingredients*

1. Take a mixing jug, add two tablespoons of coffee granules, one tablespoon of honey and mix together well.
2. Apply the delicious-smelling mixture to your face and neck, then leave for 15 minutes.
3. Rinse with lukewarm water. Your skin will feel soft and revitalized.

## *Facemask with five ingredients*

1. Mix a quarter-cup of ground oats (about half a cup of unground oats) with two to three tablespoons of warm water.
2. After 3 minutes, add two tablespoons of honey, two tablespoons of yoghurt (plain) and an egg white. Mix until the mixture is paste-like, then add a thin layer to your face.
3. Wash off after 15 minutes. Divine!

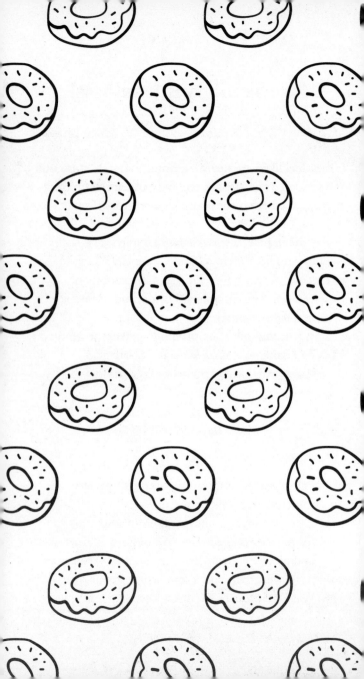

# Say 'Thank You'

Everyone likes to be appreciated, so tell someone how much you value them for something they did recently – whether they helped you through a difficult time or got you lunch when they saw you were snowed under. You may want to thank your parents, or a speaker you heard who changed the way you perceive things.

When we view life through gratitude, we experience life differently. We get to fully appreciate all the beautiful things that we otherwise take for granted. Saying 'Thank you' is beneficial to both you and the recipient – a thank-you is a win-win situation.

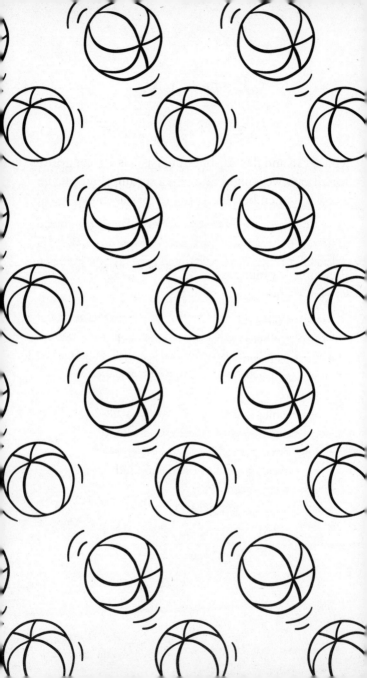

# Pasta is Life

This fresh and flavour-bursting pasta is a great go-to for an easy weeknight dinner – a scrumptious hug in a bowl. Remember: life is full of pasta-bilities.

Serves 2
Prep time – 5 minutes
Cooking time – 15–20 minutes

- 3 tbsp olive oil
- 3 large cloves garlic, finely chopped
- 2 sprigs rosemary, thyme, oregano or sage, leaves finely chopped (or 1 tsp dried)
- pinch chilli flakes
- 400g tin cherry tomatoes or passata
- 200g dried pasta
- 75g olives, artichokes or roasted red peppers from a jar, sliced
- Salt and black pepper to taste
- Parmesan or other hard cheese, to serve
- Basil leaves or chopped parsley, to serve

1. Put the kettle on to boil.
2. Heat the oil in a medium sauté or deep frying pan.
3. Add the garlic, herbs and chilli flakes and cook very gently for 2–3 minutes, until the garlic is just turning golden.
4. Tip in the cherry tomatoes or passata and squash down with a spoon, then stir in the dried pasta, olives, artichokes or peppers and some seasoning with 500ml boiling water.
5. Simmer for 15–20 minutes, stirring occasionally until the pasta is tender.
6. If using spaghetti or linguine, remember to push the pasta down into the pan as the ends soften in the sauce.
7. If the sauce is thick before the pasta is cooked, add a little more water and keep it simmering. If the sauce is too thin once the pasta is cooked, turn up the heat and bubble for 1–2 minutes, until thickened and coating the pasta.
8. Spoon into bowls and top with a generous grating of cheese and a few torn basil leaves or chopped parsley, if you like.

### Tip

- For smoky depth, fry lardons of pancetta, streaky bacon or cubes of chorizo before adding the garlic and herbs.

# Hello, World

To uplift your social battery, head out for a walk and be conscious of people around you. If you walk past somebody, try to catch their eye, smile and perhaps (gasp!) even say hello (yes, that includes you city-dwellers!). You might be surprised at how cheerful you feel when others smile or return your greetings. We are a social species, and a simple interaction can give us a massive boost of happy hormones. If you live in the sticks and there are no people around, have a chit-chat with a pigeon or a bee. Why not? Nobody will be there to hear you anyway, Dr Dolittle.

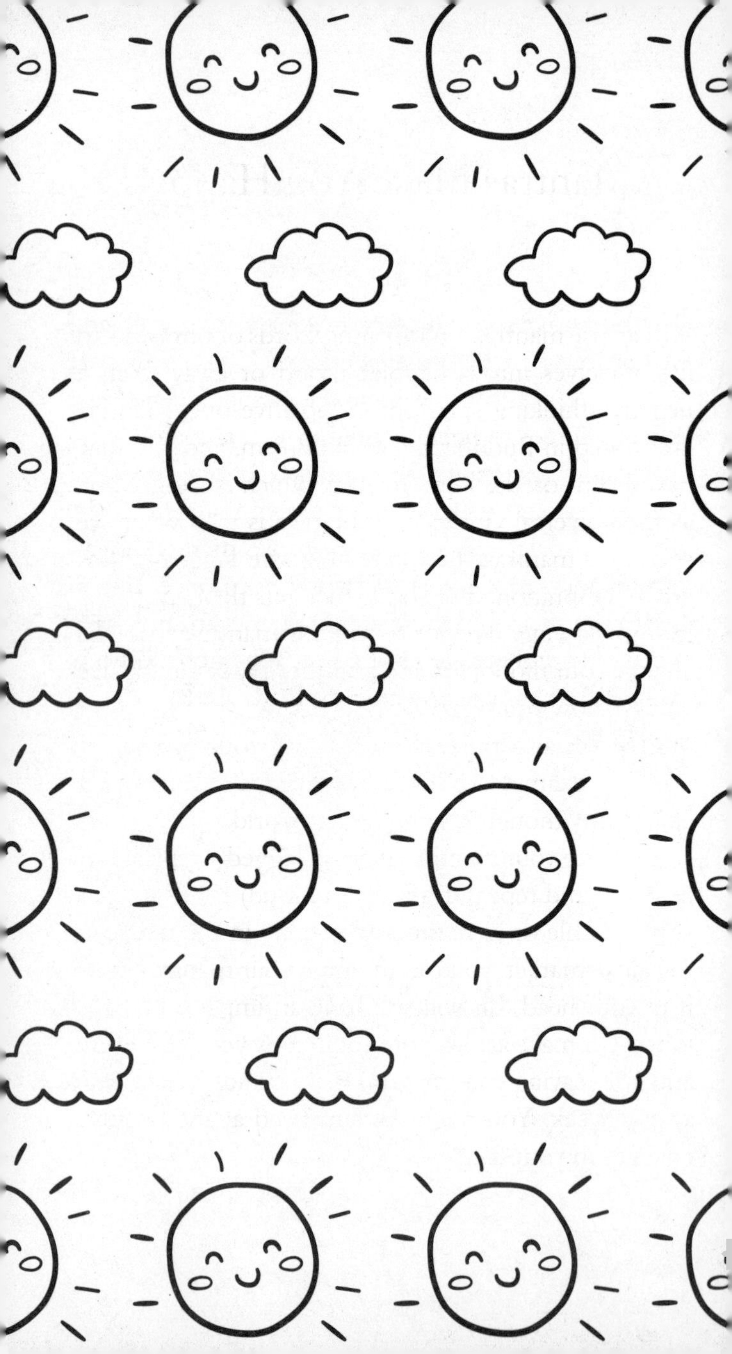

# Mantras Make You Happy!

We can use mantras – motivating words or phrases – to lift ourselves into a happier mood or away from a negative-thinking spiral into a positive one. Mantras are rooted in Buddhism and Hinduism, and you may have heard of the 'Om' mantra, which is thought of as the universal vibration. Vibration is vital when we speak of mantras. Just like when we sing, mantras create a vibration in the body that gets the happy hormones flowing. There are infinite mantras that can change your mood, life and attitude. Try some for size and see how you feel.

You can also think about writing your own mantras. An example of a simple mantra would be: 'I change my thoughts, I change my world.'

To recite your mantra, sit cross-legged on a chair or lie down and repeat it (ideally out loud) for as long as you feel able or have time. If you are in the queue at the supermarket, you can mumble your mantra or say it in your head – it will still have an impact. Perhaps journal or make a voicenote about how you feel before and after saying your mantra. Report back to yourself after a week. You might be surprised at the positive changes in your life.

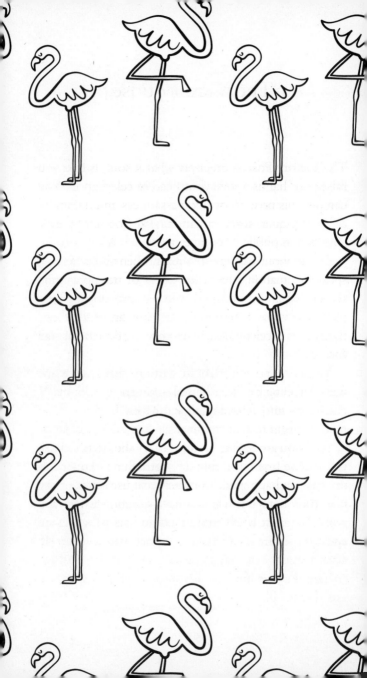

# The Victory Pose

The Victory Pose is precisely what it sounds like: you raise your hands above your head in celebration. You can use this pose to overcome sadness and deflation, or to conquer scary situations like job interviews, speaking in public or competitions.

Think about how people react when they win in a sporting situation, receive an Oscar or triumph in the school egg-and-spoon race; you will probably witness the Victory Pose: the raising of arms and fists above their heads in celebration, while bobbing the elbows – all fun stuff!

The good news is that we can use this pose when we are feeling deflated or sad and can trick the sub-conscious into releasing all the happy hormones, so that we begin to feel victorious.

So if you are having an off-day, try the Victory Pose to trick the brain into thinking something extraordinary has just happened. Another great use of this pose is to do it before you walk into a situation where you feel you might be judged or pitted against someone else. If you already feel like a winner, you will act like one.

This is a true 'fake-it-till-you-make-it' pose, and we are here for it!

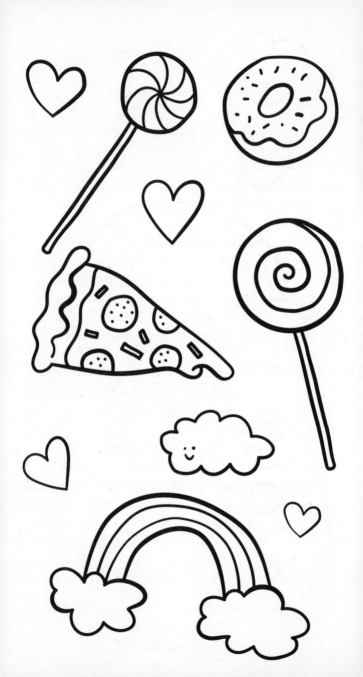

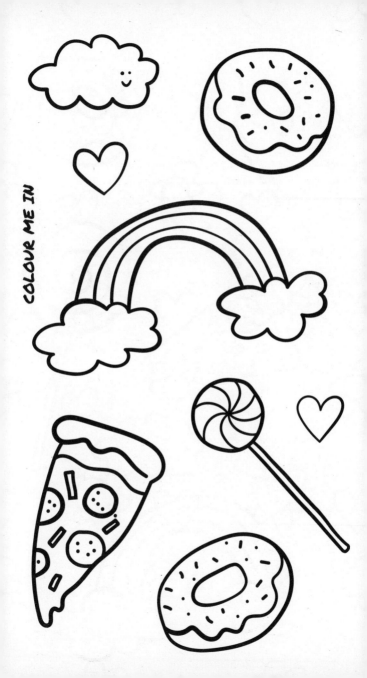

COLOUR ME IN

# The Funniest Videos on YouTube

They say that laughter is the best medicine, by helping the body relax and boosting the immune system. So if you fancy a giggle, here are some of the funniest YouTube videos to get you chuckling.

- Hysterical and Contagious Laughing Boy in Music Class
- Have You Ever Had a Dream Like This?
- 'Four Sambucas' – girl tries to order drink at DJ booth
- Dramatic Cupcake Dog – Revelation
- Lizard Jumps on Newscaster
- Zombie Kid Likes Turtles
- 'Apparently' This Kid is Awesome, Steals the Show During Interview
- Children Interrupt BBC News Interview
- Double Rainbow
- Fenton! Fenton! Fenton!
- Charlie Bit My Finger
- Dog looks at owner's plate of food and then looks away as he gets caught

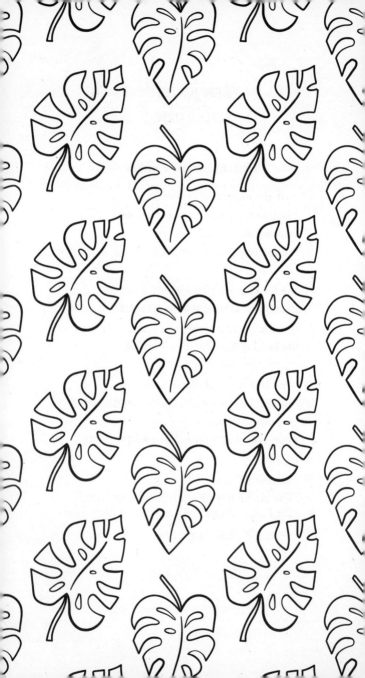

# 'Invictus'

William Ernest Henley

Out of the night that covers me,
   Black as the pit from pole to pole,
I thank whatever gods may be
   For my unconquerable soul.

In the fell clutch of circumstance
   I have not winced nor cried aloud.
Under the bludgeonings of chance
   My head is bloody, but unbowed.

Beyond this place of wrath and tears
   Looms but the Horror of the shade,
And yet the menace of the years
   Finds and shall find me unafraid.

It matters not how strait the gate,
   How charged with punishments the scroll,
I am the master of my fate,
   I am the captain of my soul.

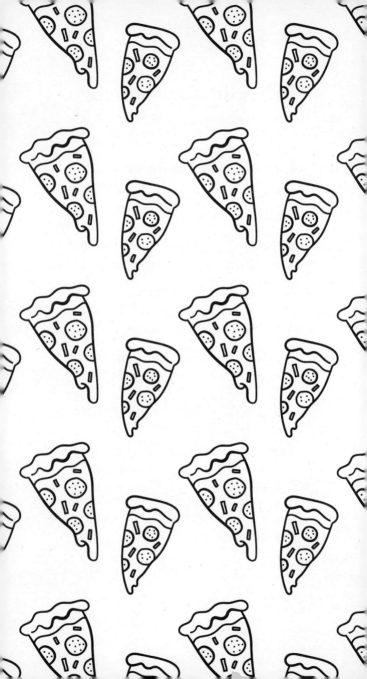

# Get Those Cogs Turning

The point of solving any puzzle is to challenge your thinking. Riddles encourage logic and problem-solving, improving concentration, focus and mental agility. To improve your capacity for critical and analytical thought, try your hand at some of these riddles. The answers are on the next page, but no peeking – you can do it!

## Questions

1. What word is pronounced the same even if you take away four of its five letters?
2. What has branches, no fruit, no trunk or leaves?
3. What do you lose the moment that you share it?
4. Two fathers and two sons are in a car, yet there are only three people in the car. How?
5. A man goes outside in the rain without an umbrella or hat, but doesn't get a single hair on his head wet. How?

ANSWERS
1. Queue  2. A bank  3. A secret  4. They are grandfather, father and son
5. The man is bald

# Energizing Breathing Exercise

Need an energy boost? Try this simple yet effective breathing technique.

1. Lie or sit somewhere comfortable.
2. Place one hand on your heart and one on your stomach.
3. Inhale through the nose for around 4 seconds, and notice your stomach rise and expand. Your stomach should press up on to your hand, and your chest should remain still.
4. Hold your breath lightly for 2 seconds.
5. Exhale steadily and slowly through your mouth for 6 seconds. Your jaw should be loose and relaxed. Notice the stomach reduction.
6. Repeat for 3–10 minutes.

If you begin to feel a little light-headed, slightly speed up your breath. Enjoy your new-found vitality!

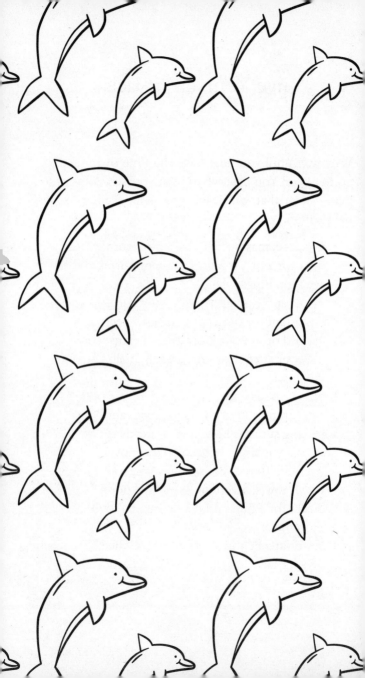

# Give Yourself a Facial

Why wait until you next have the time or money to go to a spa? You deserve to treat yourself to a pamper session that will leave your skin feeling like a baby's bum.

- **Cleanse**: massage cleanser into your face and neck for 2 or 3 minutes. Be gentle around the eye area. Rinse.
- **Tone**: apply toner with a cotton pad. Toner is important for protecting the skin because it gets rid of any stubborn dirt or extra sebum left over after cleansing, and any pollutants in the pores.
- **Steam**: pour boiled water into a large bowl and carefully hold your face 10cm above it, making sure the bowl is on a steady surface so that you don't knock the water over yourself. To trap the steam, cover your head with a towel. Steaming opens the pores. Steam for 2 minutes at a time, for a total of 10 minutes.
- **Exfoliate**: gently massage into all the corners of your face using an exfoliator, particularly

around your nose and chin, where the pores can get clogged.

- **Face mask**: Apply a sheet mask, or a home-made one (see page 83), and leave it on for 10–15 minutes, before removing it with a warm, damp cloth.
- **Apply serum**: serum stimulates collagen production, which in turn helps the skin retain its elasticity and smooth out wrinkles.
- **Eye care**: Apply your favourite eye cream by lightly tapping it on underneath and around the eye socket.
- **Moisturizing:** Apply your moisturizer thoroughly to the face, neck and upper chest. Bask in your freshness!

# Go Cloud-Spotting

Nature is everywhere – even in cities (especially the sky!). So for a moment remember how beautiful the planet is and, while walking, look up and take in the wonders of Mother Earth.

If it looks like a cloud and moves like a cloud, is it a cloud? Yes, but not all clouds are the same – there are more than 100 types. Here are the three main types you might encounter while cloud-gazing.

- **Cumulus** clouds are fluffy and white, like cotton wool, with a flat base and tops like cauliflowers. They move unhurriedly across the sky and, because they don't produce rain, are known as 'fair-weather clouds'.
- **Stratocumulus** clouds can be bright white or dark grey and are the most prevalent on Earth. They are particularly common in the UK, being spotted usually in an overcast sky when the clouds are low. They can produce light rain or snow.
- **Cumulonimbus** clouds are known more commonly as 'thunderclouds' and are the only cloud type that produces thunder, lightning and hail. They are dense, towering and typically vertical, with a hanging part that can appear to touch the ground.

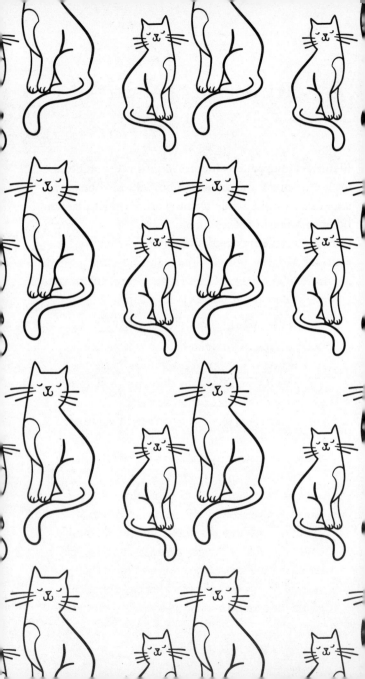

# Try Reciting a Mantra

Mantras are used as a method to calm the mind and let go of stress and anxiety. They can be a string of sounds or can be made up of words with deep symbolic meaning. They are meant to be repeated, either out loud or silently in one's thoughts. Here are some to try.

### *'I am becoming everything that I came here to be'*

This mantra is a reminder that whatever happens is supposed to happen. Even though you might feel that doors are closing in front of you, you are being directed instead towards your life's true purpose.

### *'I am' affirmations*

- I am strong
- I am confident
- I am able
- I am healthy
- I am prosperous

- I am motivated
- I am grateful
- I am joy
- I am happy
- I am loved
- I am love
- I am peace
- I am safe

Add as many affirmations as you like, and seek to experience the feeling of the words as you say them. It gets easier with practice, and you can bet you will feel calmer and happier after a few rounds of the 'I am' mantra.

# Smile

Smile, smile, smile at your mind as often as
possible. Your smiling will considerably
reduce your mind's tearing tension.
– Sri Chinmoy, Indian spiritual leader

Turn that frown upside down. Smiling is a gentle and easy way to increase your positive attitude and your confidence, as it releases the hormone dopamine, which boosts happiness and can help you handle difficult situations. A smile can instantly boost your mood and reduce tension, if the day goes wrong. Smiling can also help you to avoid burnout and feel more motivated throughout long, dull days.

Smiling also improves relationships, making you more approachable and kind, attracting other people. It makes others want to befriend you, helping you to form stronger social ties. All this, in turn, can make for a happier life, which is something worth smiling about.

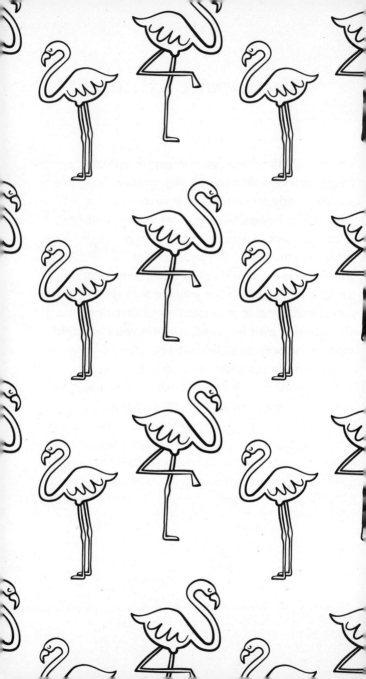

# Check In with Someone

Can you think of a friend you haven't spoken to in a long time? Or has someone you typically hear from, see frequently or who regularly posts on social media gone silent? Is someone you know behaving strangely? Why not check in with that person, if any of these are true? We often tell ourselves that we are intruding and should keep our distance, but if you push that notion aside, you could help them feel less alone and more supported. Even if you aren't feeling great yourself, you can gain a lot by assisting others, which can help put things into perspective.

If anybody came to mind while reading this, why not send them a quick 'How are you?' It has the potential to make both of your days better.

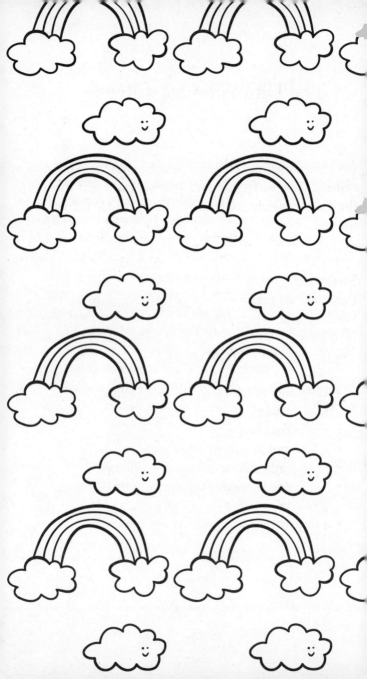

# The Ultimate Chips Recipe

Because sometimes chips are exactly what the doctor ordered. Yes, we're sure even doctors eat them when the time feels right, and they definitely couldn't say no to these ones . . .

Serves 4
Prep time – 5 minutes
Cooking time – 25 minutes

## *Ingredients*

- 1kg floury potatoes, such as Maris Piper or King Edward
- 2 tbsp cornflour
- 1 tsp smoked paprika (optional)
- ½ tsp garlic salt or onion salt (optional)
- ½ tsp dried oregano, thyme or rosemary (optional)
- 4 tbsp vegetable, sunflower or rapeseed oil

1. Heat the oven to 250°C/230°C fan/gas 9, and line two large baking trays with baking paper. Peel the potatoes and cut them into batons about 1.5cm thick.
2. Tip into a microwave-proof bowl, cover and microwave for 3 minutes on high.
3. Mix the cornflour with the seasoning and the dried spices and herbs, if using.
4. Add the microwaved batons and toss to coat.
5. Drizzle over the oil and mix again.
6. Spread the chips out on two trays and bake for 20–25 minutes, flipping them with a spatula every 5–10 minutes.
7. Serve with your favourite dipping sauce.

## Tips

- Make the chips cheesy – grate over a large handful of Cheddar and return to the oven for 1–2 minutes to melt.
- Microwaving the chips before baking helps make them crunchy outside and fluffy inside. If you don't have a microwave, blanch the batons in boiling water for 3 minutes, drain, then spread them out on tea towels to steam-dry, before coating in the flour mix.

# The Cup Song

The Cup Song (otherwise known as the Cup Game) is a craze that has swept the internet, schools and homes. When it was featured in the 2012 film *Pitch Perfect*, to the song 'When I'm Gone' by the Carter Family, it enjoyed a worldwide resurgence. Another famous Cup Game cover is 'Royals' by Lorde, covered by Sarah Stone (check it out on YouTube – it's brilliant!).

## *You will need*

- A plastic or paper cup

## *How to do the intro to the Cup Song from* Pitch Perfect

1. Clap twice above the cup. **Clap-Clap**.
2. Tap on the cup three times, using a different hand each time. **Right – Tap, Left – Tap, Right – Tap**.
3. **Clap**.

4. Pick up the cup with your right hand and move to the right. **Pick Up and Move Right**.
5. **Clap**.
6. Put it all together. **Clap-Clap, Tap, Tap, Tap, Clap, Pick Up and Move Right, Clap**.

Hey presto, a new party trick!

# Feel-Good News: Some good spud news!

In November 2022 findings were reported that potatoes can help you lose weight. Potatoes were long thought too 'starchy' to be a diet food; however, a study in the US showed that they can help people lose weight without increasing glucose.

Thirty-six participants, aged 18 to 60, were either overweight or obese and were put on diets rich in vegetables, with 40 per cent of the usual meat content replaced with beans and peas or potatoes (including wedges!). Over two months, the potato-eaters lost the same weight as the pea- and bean-eaters.

The main reason was that as potatoes were more filling, people ate less of them, thus efficiently reducing the number of calories.

Mash for dinner tonight?

(www.theweek.co.uk)

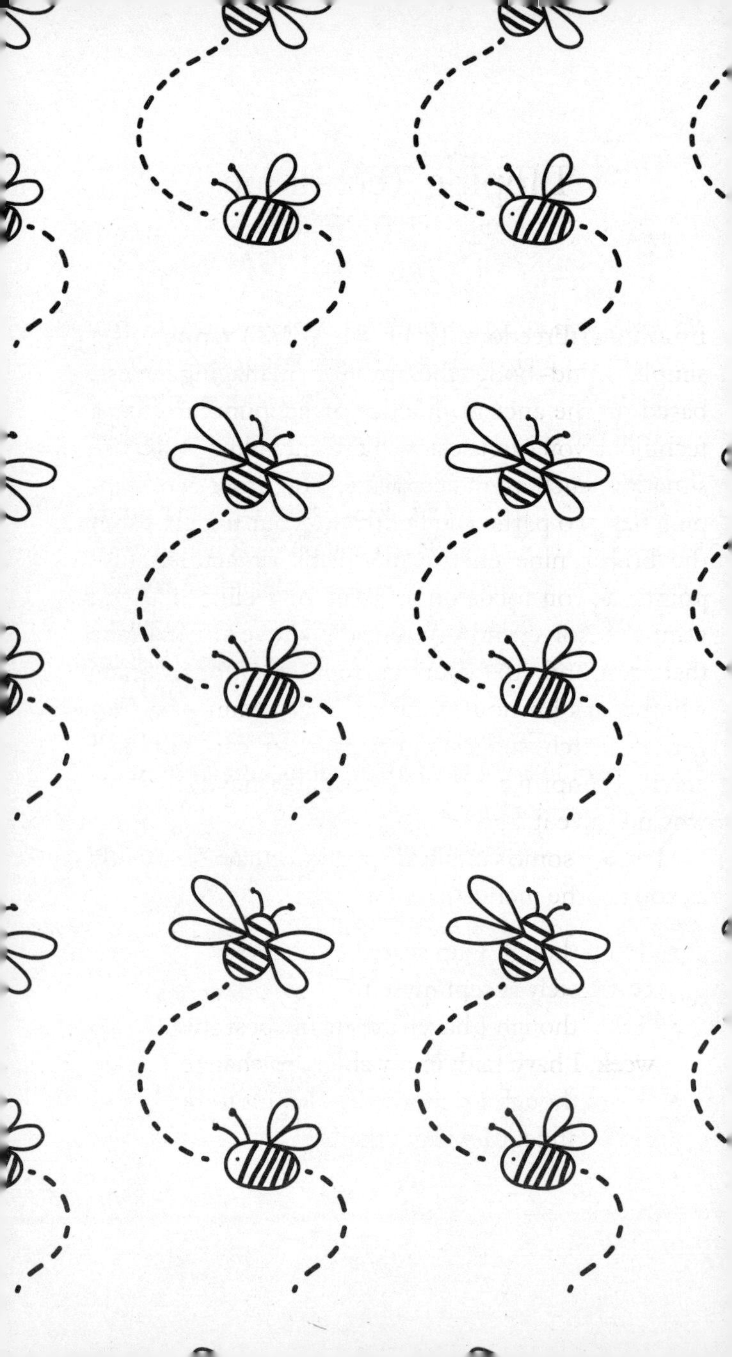

# Tapping Technique

Emotional Freedom Technique (EFT) tapping is a simple mind–body therapy for managing stress, based on the ancient practice of acupuncture. It's a technique you can use anywhere, including in a tense situation, such as an aeroplane. The process of tapping has two parts: you lightly tap your fingertips on the body's nine energy meridians or acupuncture points, as you focus on an issue or feeling that you want to resolve; and you repeat positive affirmations that respond to your current emotional state, whether it's burnout, sadness, anger, pain or a trigger. Research suggests that tapping can diminish cravings, improve performance and relieve stress, so why not give it a go?

Here are some sample affirmations that you can say as you tap the meridians:

- 'Even though I am scared to be myself, I completely accept myself.'
- 'Even though I haven't done my best this week, I have faith in my ability to change.'
- 'Even though I'm not where I want to be, I am confident I will get there.'

Here are the nine meridians or acupuncture points to move through as you tap with your fingertips and repeat your affirmation three times:

1. Karate chop – the outer edge of both hands, where the flesh is thicker
2. Eyebrow – between your eyebrows, at the start at the top of your nose
3. Side of the eyes – on the bone around the outside of either eye
4. Under the eyes – on top of the cheekbone under either eye
5. Under the nose – between the nose and upper lip
6. Chin – between your bottom lip and chin
7. The collarbone – just below where your collarbones meet, about 5cm apart
8. Under the arm – about 10cm under each armpit
9. Top of the head – directly on the crown of your head

# Fridge Cake

Everyone loves fridge cake because you can make it in minutes, it looks impressive and tastes great. Give it a try and dazzle your guests (or yourself – you deserve it!).

Serves 9–12
Prep time – 10 minutes plus chilling
Cooking time – 5 minutes

- 100g marshmallows
- 100g butter
- 100g toffees or chewy caramels
- 185g puffed rice or cornflakes
- 250g milk or dark chocolate
- 25g white chocolate (optional)
- Sprinkles or chopped-up chocolate bars to decorate (optional)

1. Butter and line a 20cm-deep round cake tin or square brownie tin with baking paper.
2. Melt the marshmallows, butter and toffees or caramels in a large saucepan, stirring often.
3. Remove from the heat, tip in the cereal and stir until well coated.

4. Scrape into the tin and press down with the back of a spoon to fill any gaps.
5. Melt the milk or dark chocolate in a heatproof bowl over a pan of gently simmering water, or in 30-second bursts on low in the microwave.
6. Pour the chocolate over the cake. If using, melt the white chocolate, then drizzle over the top, for a marble effect.
7. Scatter over sprinkles or chopped-up chocolate to decorate, if you like.
8. Chill for about 30 minutes until set, then slice and serve.

# Have a Cuddle

One of the best ways to boost our happy hormones is to give or receive a hug. Everyone loves a cuddle, right? Well, no, not everyone – and that's fair enough. However, you only live once, and even if you don't consider yourself a hugger, why not surprise your bestie with a big bear hug the next time you see them? You might be surprised at how bonded and happy you feel in that moment (that's the oxytocin release, but let's not get technical and ruin the moment!).

If no one else is around for a cuddle, feel free to throw your arms around yourself and give yourself a big squeeze. You could even say 'Thank you' for all the times you've done nice things for yourself, smile and take a deep breath. So give it a go; the chances are it will feel great.

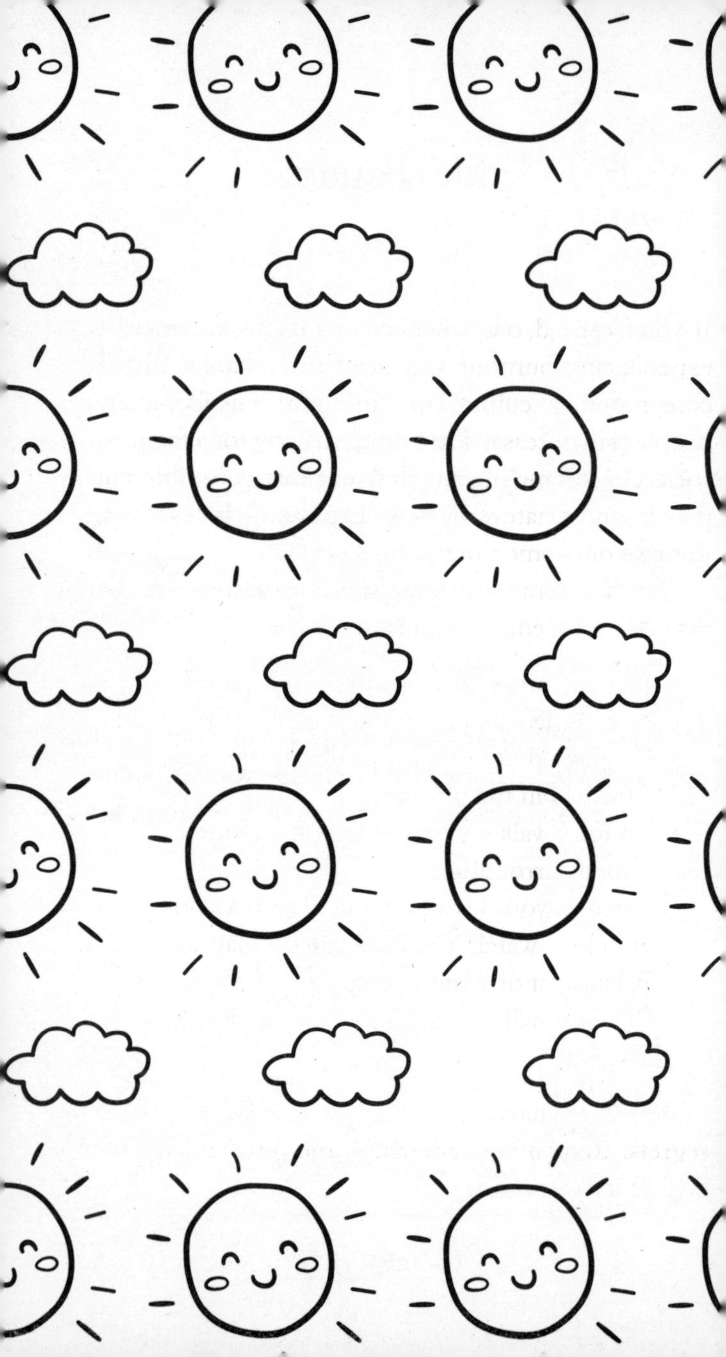

# Me-Time

If you feel tired, overwhelmed or anxious, you may be experiencing burnout and need to recharge. In the contemporary culture of 'the side hustle', many people skip necessary 'me-time', making for a fatigued society. 'Me-time' means different things to different people, and whatever it looks like to you, it's essential to carve out some time for it.

Here are some great 'me-time' suggestions to get the 'ahh' moments you truly deserve.

- Take the pressure off yourself and cancel your immediate plans, if you can.
- Get a good night's sleep and wake up refreshed in the morning.
- Go for a walk and pay attention to your natural surroundings.
- Listen to your favourite music, read a book, sit in bed, watch YouTube videos, play an instrument or write a story.
- Get your nails done, take a bath or visit a museum.

Whatever makes you tick, go and do it with no regrets. Remember: adequate 'me-time' makes for healthier 'we-time'.

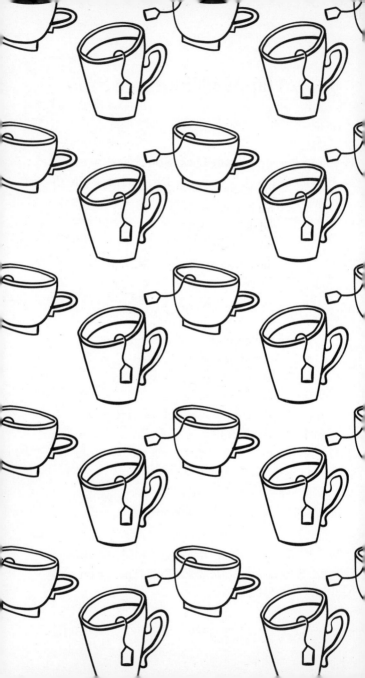

# 'How Happy is the Little Stone'

## Emily Dickinson

How happy is the little stone
That rambles in the road alone,
And doesn't care about careers,
And exigencies never fears;
Whose coat of elemental brown
A passing universe put on;
And independent as the sun,
Associates or glows alone,
Fulfilling absolute decree
In casual simplicity.

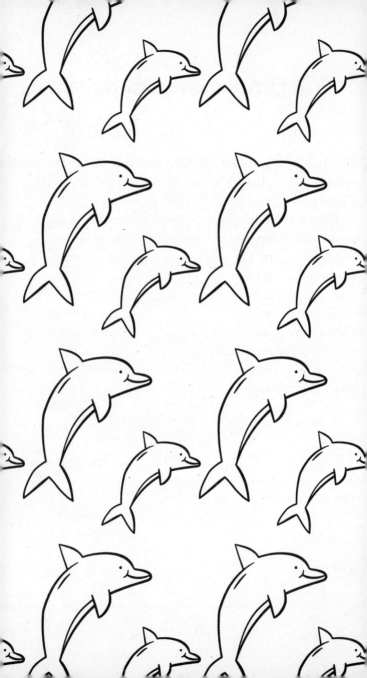

# Run Around the Block

This run is aptly named for those who live near a convenient 'block', but it's just as effective to run around a local park, if you have one close to home.

Motivating yourself for a quick run after a long day at work is challenging, but the positive effects far outweigh the effort. The point of this exercise is not to reach any 5–10-kilometre milestones; it's simply to clear away the cobwebs and get your heartbeat pumping; running gives us a great kick of feel-good endorphins, known as a 'runner's high'. Afterwards you can bet that you will feel more motivated to complete other tasks, cook healthier meals and will sleep much better at night.

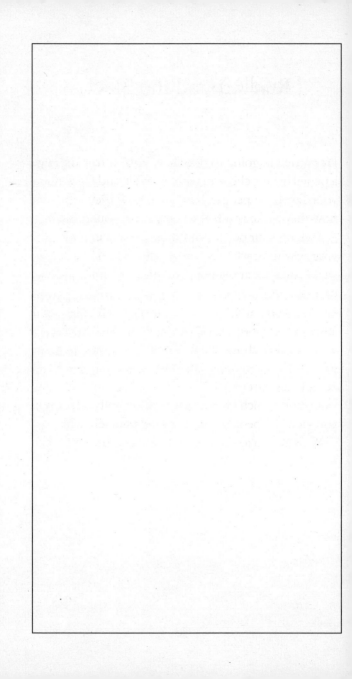

# Doodle Your Best Friends

Here you are going to doodle your best friends. Have a pencil handy, check in with yourself and think about your favourite people. Think of how they look, and how they make you feel when you're around them.

Pick up your pencil with those people in mind. Ask your intuition: what do these people look like? What shape or size are they? Are these people tall, well dressed, funny, happy or serious?

Simply begin drawing on the opposite page or in another notebook and allow your hand to express the way you feel about them. Then when you have finished, take a moment to look at the drawing and accept it as part of you. This offers your subconscious validation, which gives you an opportunity to see how you view the people you surround yourself with.

We dare you to share your drawing with your friends!

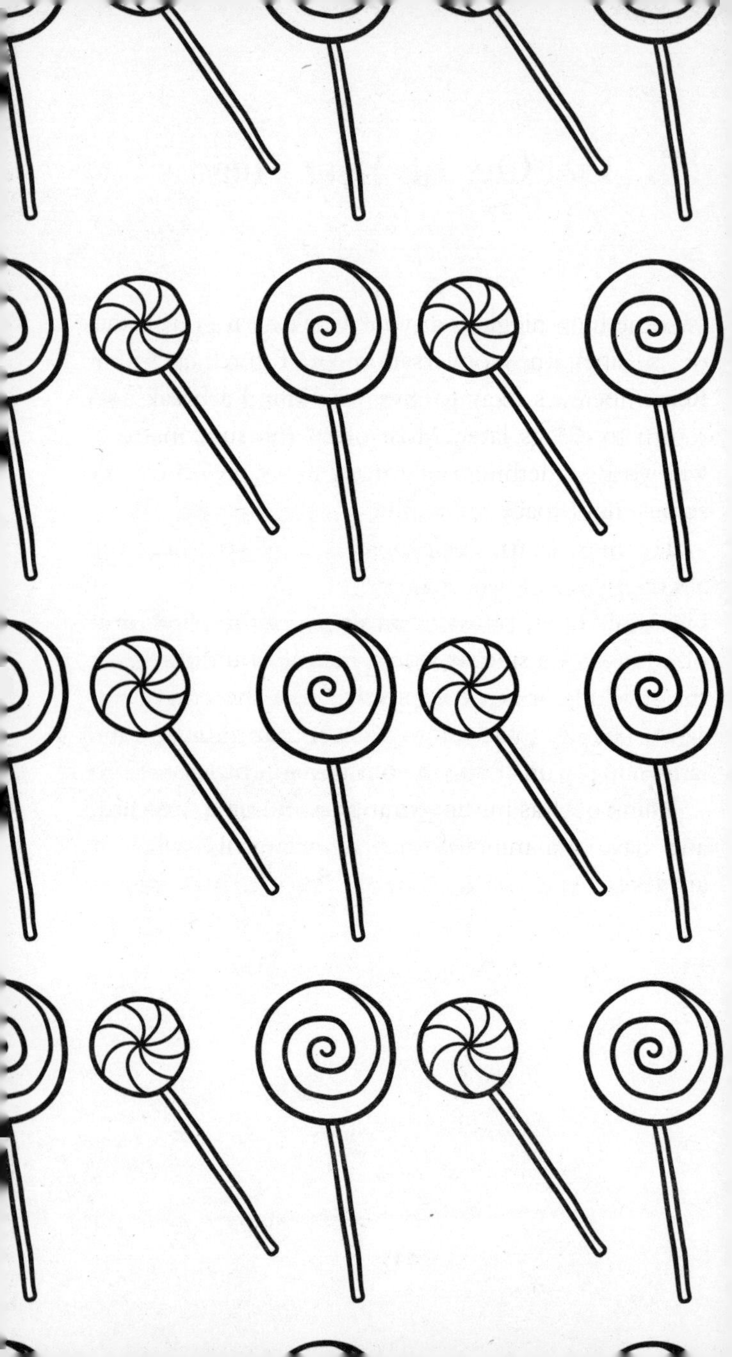

# Get Out of Your Head

Is something niggling at you? Can't clear your mind of a situation, conversation or future decision? Remember: it's okay to give your mind a break and return to things later. Most often the subconscious will work something out for us, if we give the conscious mind space to breathe.

Try this trick to get a problem out of your head for a while. Write down whatever is bothering you on a piece of paper, put it in an envelope or a box and place it to one side. It would help if you didn't hide the envelope or box completely, but it shouldn't be in sight. That way, you know you can return to the issue later, and it won't cling to your thought processes.

Think of it as putting your problem on a postcard, and have the mindset that 'It will arrive when it arrives'.

# Joke: An Empty Seat

It's the World Cup Final, and a man makes his way to his seat next to the pitch. He sits down and notices that the seat next to him is empty. So he leans over and asks the stranger on the other side of the seat if someone will sit there.

'No,' says the stranger. 'The seat is vacant.'

'This is incredible,' says the man, 'who in their right mind would buy this seat for the World Cup Final and not use it?'

'Well, actually,' the stranger says, 'the seat belongs to me. I was supposed to be here with my wife, but she passed away. In fact, this is the first World Cup Final we haven't attended together since we got married.'

'Oh, I'm so sorry to hear that; that's so sad. Surely you could find someone else – a relative, friend or even a neighbour – to come with you, though?'

The man shakes his head. 'No,' he says. 'They're all at the funeral.'

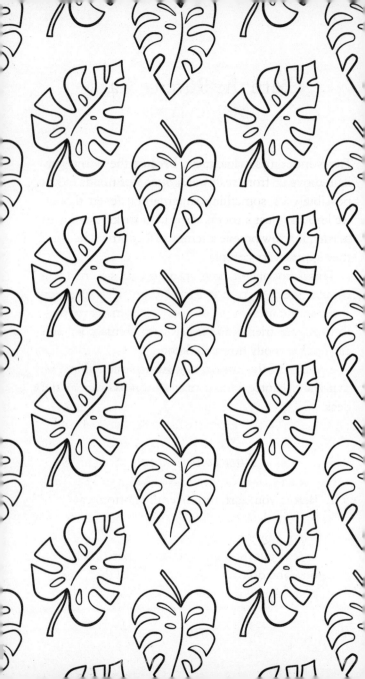

# Learn the Reverse Card
# Magic Trick

Everyone enjoys magic tricks, because they temporarily remove us from reality and open our minds to the possibility of something supernatural (even though we know it's just a trick). Many card tricks are easy to master, but few people attempt to learn them because they appear very complex.

This is not one of them. Here is your sign that you should give it a go; it is fun to learn (if you have a spare 10 minutes), and you have a lifetime party trick to wow your friends and family with. Remember: you can't tell anybody how you did it!

The aim of this trick is to make the audience think that the volunteer's card magically flips over in the deck.

## How to perform it

1. Before you start, turn over the bottom card of your deck (secretly), so it's the only card facing upwards.
2. Spread out the cards and let the person pick one, and do your best not to reveal the bottom card that you have faced up. Tell the

volunteer to remember their card and to show it to everyone else but you.

3. While they do this, turn the cards in your hands over casually. This should leave all the cards, except the top one, facing up in your left hand.

4. Put the spectator's chosen card face-down in the middle of the deck and keep it tight, to hide the fact that the cards are back to front.

5. Put the cards behind your back and tell them you'll find their card without looking. While you're doing so, turn the top card over (secretly), so that it is facing up.

6. Take the face-up cards and fan through them until you find the only face-down card. *Voilà*: impress the room by showing the volunteer's chosen card.

Search for this on YouTube – Card Magic Trick: Their Card Reversed in the Deck! – for a more in-depth tutorial.

That's magic!

# Dreamy Hot Chocolate

Believe it or not, flavonoids, which increase blood flow, are abundant in hot chocolate. Improved blood flow to the brain decreases the risk of blood clots, lowers blood pressure, enhances heart health and helps you think more clearly. So, come rain or shine, this dreamy hot chocolate is guaranteed to put a smile on your face.

Serves 1, or more depending on how much milk you use
Prep time – 5 minutes

- A bar of chocolate (milk or dark)
- Dairy or soy milk (enough for the number of cups you want to serve)
- Sugar (to taste)
- Topping ideas: whipped cream, marshmallows, grated chocolate

1. Cut the bar of chocolate into small chunks, place them on a plate and microwave until melted.
2. Heat the milk in a saucepan and add a sprinkle of sugar if you like (best for dark chocolate).

3. Over a medium heat, bring the milk to around 82°C. To know when you're at this temperature, look for tiny bubbles beginning to form on the sides of the saucepan before it boils. Try not to boil the milk.

4. Turn off the heat when the milk is hot and add the melted chocolate while stirring it into the milk.

5. Whisk until frothy and serve in your favourite cup/mug.

6. Add your toppings of choice: marshmallows and whipped cream are perfect for an extra-tasty treat.

# Get Dressed Up

If you have a job that requires you to dress up, then sitting around in your pyjamas or comfortable clothes all day can be a huge luxury. However, dressing up *just* because you feel like it can be an excellent boost for your confidence.

Put on your favourite outfit that makes you feel like a million dollars. Then do your hair and make-up so that you feel your most glamorous. You always deserve to feel great, even if you aren't going anywhere. You don't have to wait for the outside world to see you looking your best: do it for yourself.

Getting dressed up is also a great trick if you want to go out, but are feeling lazy and lack motivation. Here's betting you're more likely to step out of the door once you feel your best.

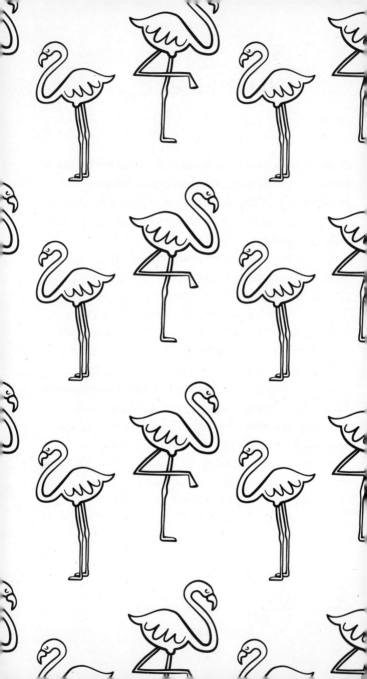

# Riddle Me This . . .

Riddles are a great way to practise your lateral thinking and get the cogs turning. They are also said to boost memory speed and improve concentration so, whether you need a 5-minute distraction at your desk or want to get people talking at your next dinner party, give this one a go. The answer is on the following page, but give yourself some time to ponder before peeking!

## *Question*

A man wants to enter a private club, but he doesn't know the password. He watches a woman walk up to the doorman who says '12', she responds '6' and is let in. Another man walks up to the entrance, the doorman says '6', the man says '3', and is let in. Thinking he's figured it out, he walks up to the door and the doorman says '10', he confidently replies '5', but is turned away. What should he have said?

## *Answer*

Three – the code is the number of letters that are in the number the doorman says.

# Put Together a Care Package

Why not join the many people who have put together care packages for people in Ukraine who have lost their homes? Millions around the world have gathered and transported all sorts of commodities, including non-perishable food, toys, clothes, medical equipment and other items, for immediate use by volunteers and relief organizations. If you want to take the same action, group the items you want to send by category, list what each box contains and identify the items as 'Humanitarian aid' while assembling care packages.

Visit this link – helpukraine.center/#send-aid – to learn what it would be most useful to send, and where to send your box. Or go to the Disasters Emergency Committee website (dec.org.uk) for other ways to support those in need.

Alternatively, if you have old clothes that you no longer need, you can donate them to the British Red Cross by post for free, to be sold in their shops to raise funds for all the work they do in responding to crises and supporting people around the world. Just head to: giftshop.redcross.org.uk/products/donate-by-post.

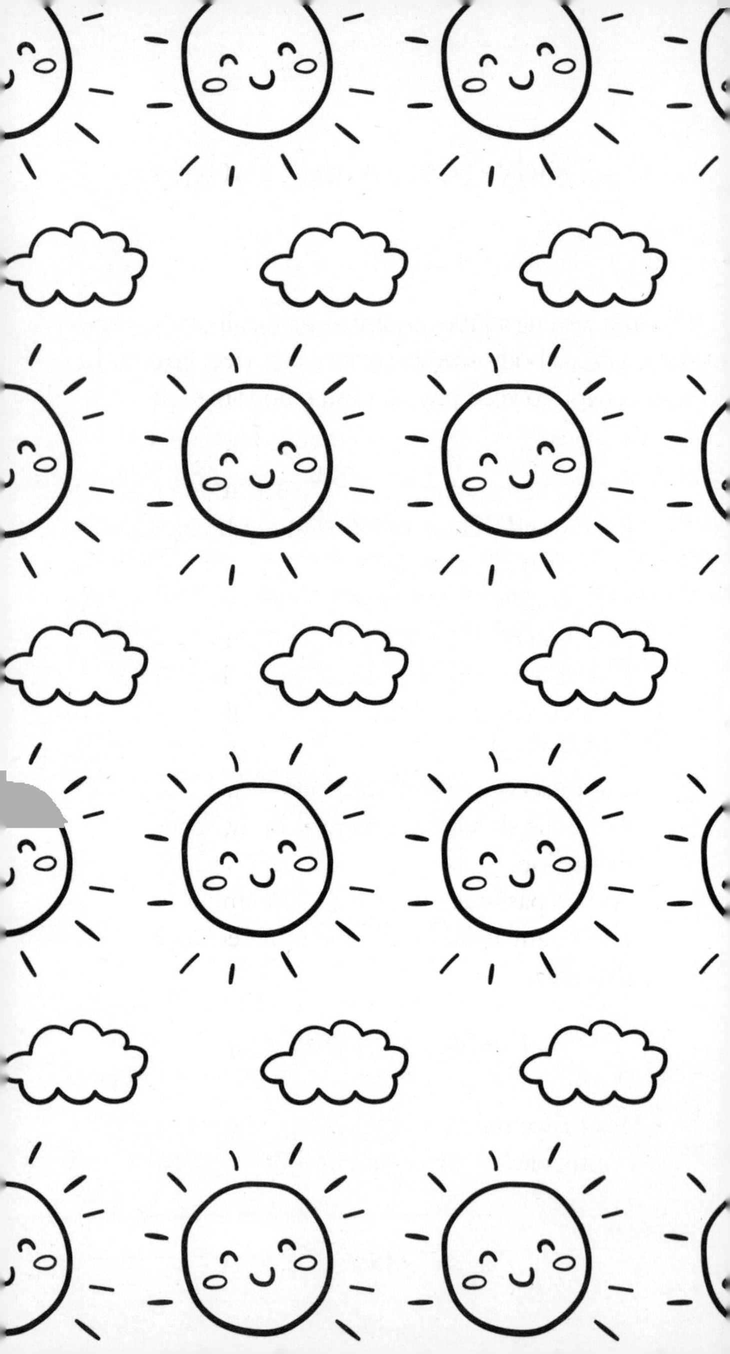

# Body-Scan Meditation

If you're feeling a little disjointed, as we all do now and then, a quick body-scan exercise is a perfect remedy to connect you to your physical and emotional self.

1. Find a comfortable resting position.
2. Take 10 grounding breaths by breathing in deeply and sighing out. Counting the breaths helps you to focus and relax.
3. Start your body-scan by placing your attention on the top (crown) of your head and observe any sensations. Focus here for 20–30 seconds and breathe naturally.
4. Next, in your mind, focus on your forehead and observe the area with curiosity.
5. Continue slowly scanning the body, section by section.
6. As you pass each body part, remember to release any tension you might be feeling in that area.

### *A guide on areas to scan*

- Head area: the crown, forehead, cheeks, jaw, mouth, back of head and neck

- Shoulders, elbows, lower arms and hands (one side of the body at a time)
- Torso/mid-body: the chest (front and back), lungs, heart, spine (going down vertebra by vertebra), belly, lower back, pelvis and hips
- Upper legs, knees, lower legs, feet (one side of the body at a time)

Remember to bring compassion and non-judgemental awareness to each body part that you observe. After you complete the body-scan, take a few big, deep breaths. Then, as with other meditations, be patient and accept your experience. With practice, the body-scan should immediately begin to ground and connect you.

# Press Some Flowers

Pressing flowers is one of those rewarding activities that requires minimal effort, but is a beautiful way to remember a point in time – be it a woodland walk with a loved one, a wedding or a gift from someone special. If you don't have any flowers around the house or garden right now, why not head out on a walk to pick some; you'll be surprised what you can find!

## *How to make your flower press*

1. Choose flowers that are almost in full bloom.
2. Make sure the flowers are as dry as possible.
3. If a flower's petals are layered (like a rose), take them apart before pressing them and you can put them back together afterwards.
4. The best (amateur) way to press flowers is in a book and, of course, the heavier and sturdier the book, the better. The alternative way is to buy a professional flower press, which isn't too expensive and is definitely worth investing in, if you want to refine the creative process.

5. Use paper around the flowers to absorb moisture. You can use blotting paper, tissue or paper towels, cardboard or newspaper. Use between three and twelve sheets to absorb the moisture effectively.
6. Do not disturb the flowers during the drying process, which will take approximately two to three weeks.
7. Weight down the drying 'chamber' – this means putting a brick or a heavy stone on top of the book.

Afterwards you can remove your flowers and arrange them in a frame; use them in a collage, to bring your memory to life with words, photos and drawings; or create an album of your beautiful flower pressings, with annotations to remind you where they came from.

# Give Yourself a Head Massage

Giving yourself a soothing head massage can relieve tension, headaches and stress, so it's a great thing to learn how to do this yourself!

## *How to do it*

1. You can start by standing, sitting or lying down – whichever works in the moment. Gently apply pressure on the area around the temples with your knuckles.
2. Extend your fingers and use the tips to move in gentle, circular strokes in the same area.
3. Begin to move up to the scalp region, and spend at least 5 minutes here, moving the fingertips in a circular motion.
4. Afterwards start massaging at the nape of the neck, just below the scalp. Work your way down to relieve stress in the shoulder and collarbone area.
5. Next put your left hand between your right shoulder and the right side of your neck, where there is usually a lot of tension, and massage; then switch sides and repeat this cycle.

6. Finally hold your head in the palms of your hands (fingers facing towards the crown), as if you were holding a football, and apply pressure. Release and feel the tension fade away.
7. Once you have finished, close your eyes and relax for 15 minutes.

# Banana Smoothie

Bananas are known as the 'happy fruit' because they contain the amino acid 'tryptophan', which transforms into serotonin in the body. Serotonin lifts your mood, calms you down and makes you happier. (Also, because bananas are rich in potassium, they are one of the best hangover cures on the planet!) The best part, though, is that they are delicious! So, with all that said, here is how to make the *perfect* banana smoothie.

Serves 2
Prep time – 5 minutes

- 2 ripe bananas, peeled and chopped
- 375ml (1½ cups) skimmed milk
- 70g (¼ cup) low-fat natural yoghurt
- 1 tbsp honey
- 4–6 ice cubes

1. Put the bananas in a blender, along with the milk, yoghurt, honey and ice. Blend until well mixed.
2. Serve in glasses. Add extra honey on top to taste.

Thanks for attending today's sundae school.

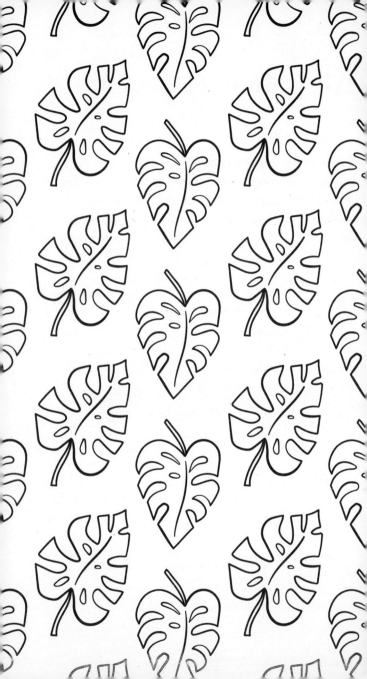

# Go Tree-Hunting

When we are out and about, we get so distracted that we forget to be present and appreciate nature. So the next time you are out in the world, make it your mission to look out for at least one of these trees.

## *Silver birch*, Betula pendula

This is a striking and medium-sized deciduous tree that can reach nine metres in height and be identified by its papery white bark, which sheds like layers of tissue paper, leaving a black and rugged base. Its elegant branches droop, forming a light canopy, and its leaves are triangular with toothed (jagged) edges and pointed tips.

## *Oak tree*, Quercus robur

The oak is often referred to when describing something old and robust. Slow-growing from a tiny sapling, it can take up to 100 years before it reaches full stature, and can live for up to 500 years in an ideal growing location. It's identifiable by its famous seed – the acorn – and its leaves have between two and five lobes (you can think of them as leaf fingers).

## *Horse chestnut*, Aesculus hippocastanum

This is one of the most common and well-known trees, due to its famous seed offering: the conker! As autumn descends and the spiky green husk falls from the trees, the shiny brown conker begins to emerge. The horse chestnut has a broad and tall trunk, with palmate (hand-shaped) leaves with five to seven 'toothed' (jagged) 'leaflets' (a leaf-like part of a compound leaf).

# Write a Limerick

Writing a limerick is creative, fun and can be as profound or as juvenile as you like. The rules are simple: the first, second and fifth lines all rhyme with one another (we'll call these 'A rhymes'), and the third and fourth lines must rhyme with each other (we'll call these 'B rhymes').

We now have an AABBA rhyme scheme ('Mamma Mia'!), and the format looks like this:

- Line 1 – **A** (8–9 syllables)
- Line 2 – **A** (8–9 syllables)
- Line 3 – **B** (5–6 syllables)
- Line 4 – **B** (5–6 syllables)
- Line 5 – **A** (8–9 syllables)

Here are a couple of examples to get you started. Remember, you can draw inspiration from anywhere: your pets, office, family or favourite science fact; just give it a whirl and get your creative juices flowing!

> There was a young schoolboy of Rye,
> Who was baked by mistake in a pie.
> To his mother's disgust,
> He emerged through the crust,
> And exclaimed, with a yawn, 'Where am I?'

Or:

A creature of charm is the gerbil.
Its diet's exclusively herbal.
It grazes all day,
On bunches of hay,
Passing gas with a loud burble.

# Try These Ancient Mantras

A mantra, which is a repeated word or phrase, can be used as a tool for letting go of thoughts. Chanting mantras can have a significant impact on you, especially if you struggle with focus and mental preparation. People who use mantras regularly report that it helps them become more self-aware and sharpens their focus. Try the following mantras and see if you feel differently afterwards.

## Hari om

This mantra is believed to erase all suffering and connect those who use it with universal consciousness ('om'). *Hari* in Sanskrit means 'the remover' or 'the one who takes away'. Therefore chanting 'Hari om' can give your life a cleansing of negativity and can invite happiness and prosperity into it.

## Om mani padme hum

The literal meaning in English is 'praise to the jewel in the lotus'. However, this mantra does not have a direct translation. Instead it's said that each syllable symbolizes one of the six internal forces that cause suffering: jealousy, desire, ego, hate, prejudice and possessiveness. Therefore saying this mantra helps replace these feelings with those of patience, generosity, ethics, concentration, perseverance and wisdom.

# Sort Your Drawers

It's true that a tidy house equals a tidy mind, so what does your underwear drawer say about your state of mind? If you have been avoiding this task for a long time, don't fret! We are here with good news: if you do it correctly just *one* time, it is guaranteed to make you feel calmer and more in control as you start each day – that's the aim anyway!

Investing in a drawer organizer will make this a dream job. By having a place for different styles and colours, you can more easily navigate to whichever item you need and help keep your drawers tidy for good. However, before that, it's important to sort your underwear and/or socks into these piles:

| I wear often | I might wear again | I will never wear again |
| --- | --- | --- |

Be brutally honest and remove the items in the last column. The things in the first column go to the front of your drawer, and the middle column is neatly folded and put nearer the back. This may seem like a 'teaching you to suck eggs' suggestion, but if you haven't had a clear-out in a while, it's time to get in there and be ruthless – be gone with that odd holey, faded sock from 2013! It's worth it – we promise.

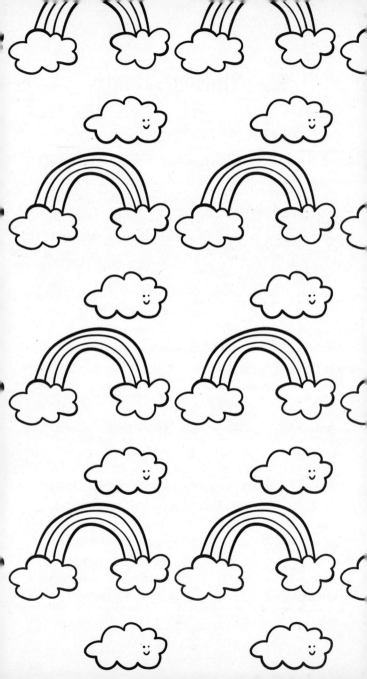

# 'Riches'

### Sara Teasdale

I have no riches but my thoughts,
Yet these are wealth enough for me;
My thoughts of you are golden coins
Stamped in the mint of memory;

And I must spend them all in song,
For thoughts, as well as gold, must be
Left on the hither side of death
To gain their immortality.

# *The* Margarita Recipe

The Margarita needs no introduction – it's the most popular cocktail in the world. It is zesty and tasty, and you can serve it in any vessel without losing any cred. So whether or not it's five o'clock, it's Margarita time.

Serves 2
Prep time – 5 mins

- Ice
- 120ml tequila
- 60ml Cointreau
- 60ml lime juice
- 15ml agave syrup or honey
- Sea salt
- Lime peel (for the glass)
- Lime wedges (to garnish)

1. Pour ice halfway into a shaker or big measuring cup.
2. Add the tequila, Cointreau, lime juice and agave syrup or honey. Shake or stir until completely cooled.

3. Pour the sea salt on to a plate, rub the lime peel round the rims of the glasses and dip the rims into the salt.
4. Add ice into the glasses before straining the Margarita over the top.
5. Add a lime wedge as garnish.

# Desk Stretches

Sitting at a desk all day can affect our mood, posture and health. Here are a few moves that you can try to alleviate desk-sitting stiffness.

## *Tilt your head*

1. Relax your neck and upper back to avoid headaches.
2. Sitting up straight, gently move your head towards one shoulder with your hand. Hold for 10–15 seconds and release; do on alternate sides.
3. To tilt your head left, gently pull on the chair's left side with your right hand. The right shoulder and neck should extend. Hold for 10–30 seconds and then switch sides.

## *Overhead stretching*

1. Press upwards with your fingers above your head for a few seconds before releasing.

2. Sit upright and reach your right arm over your head to stretch your side.
3. Then gently lean left until your right side stretches further.
4. Repeat with the left arm above your head, for 10–30 seconds.

## Chest stretch

1. Clasp your hands behind you, whether you are sitting or standing.
2. Stretch your arms and gradually elevate them until your chest stretches. Hold for 10–30 seconds.

# Ask for Help

We all need help sometimes, but often we prevent ourselves from seeking it. Maybe you view asking for help as a weakness, think you are burdening others or you're worried about being judged. You can turn those concerns around by realizing that asking for help is, in fact, a strength, and that people will be more than happy to offer help if they know you need it.

The best way to think of it is: 'How would I react if someone I cared about asked for my help?' Therein lies your answer.

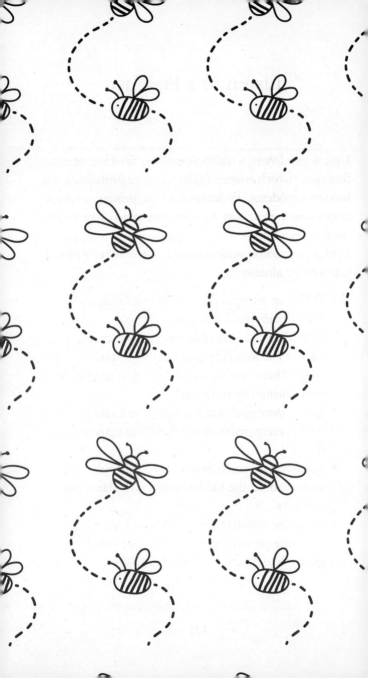

# Listen to a Podcast

Unless you live in a technology-free, Wi-Fi- and data-free cave (which sounds idyllic), you've probably got a favourite podcast. Podcasts are fun, primarily educational and a great way to keep our minds busy while we do other things.

Here are some podcasts you should check out, if you haven't already:

- *Off Menu*: an array of celebrities talking about their dream meal, presented by two comedians, Ed Gamble and James Acaster
- *How to Fail with Elizabeth Day*: an inspiring listen where celebrities talk about what they have learned from failure
- *Script Apart*: each week a movie buff chats with screenwriters about their first screenplay drafts
- *Unearthed: Mysteries from an Unseen World*: stories about the hidden impact of plants on our lives
- *Serial*: the ultimate true-crime podcast, which has gone on to inspire hundreds of other greats, like *West Cork* and *Sweet Bobby*

- *You're Dead to Me*: episodes on key figures and periods in history, which you should know about, but have probably forgotten since school
- *Sh\*\*ged, Married, Annoyed*: comedian Chris Ramsey and his wife, Rosie, talk about anything and everything that has bothered them that week

# Feel-Good News: Brothers who were neighbours

Soon after birth, brothers Tommy Larkin and Stephen Goosney were adopted by separate families. Goosney was raised in Woody Point on Newfoundland's North Peninsula, while Larkin grew up 200 kilometres north.

When both brothers were 29 years old, they independently decided to look for one another through a post-adoption agency. They were handed news that neither of them were expecting – they had been living opposite one another on the same street for two years!

They got along like a house on fire and spent the following summer having back-garden barbecues and catching up on an entire lifetime.

(myheritage.com)

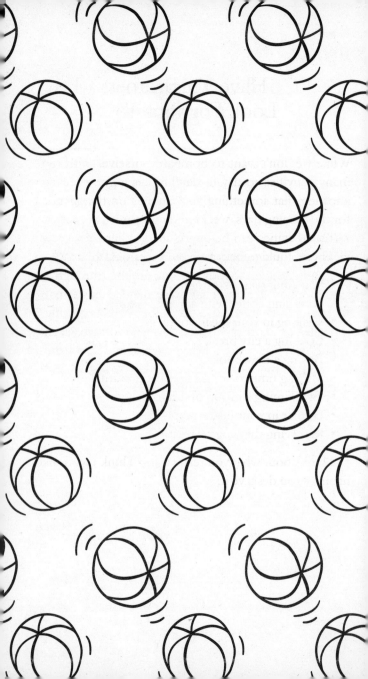

# Have Things to Look Forward To

While we don't want to bombard ourselves with too many activities in day-to-day life, it's a great feeling knowing that something you enjoy is on the agenda for the coming days, weeks and months.

The activities can be big or small – here are a few ideas you could pencil into your 'happy calendar':

- Watching your favourite film
- Grabbing coffee with a good friend
- Walking in your local woodland
- Booking a city break
- Buying a new book
- Making time to sit, drink tea and journal
- FaceTiming a group of friends
- Dinner in your nearest city
- Reserving that yoga retreat

Think about what you really want. Think big, think happy – you deserve it.

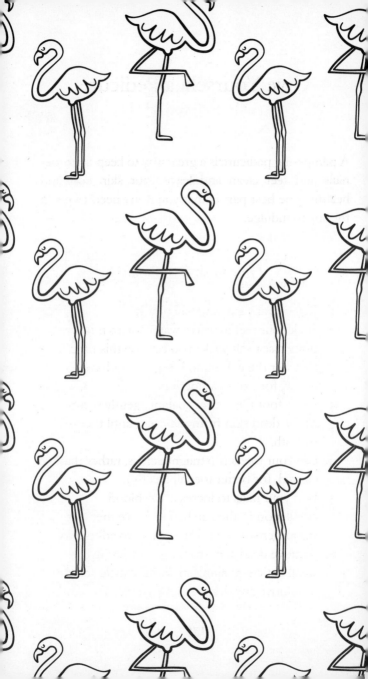

# Give Yourself a Pedicure

A pampering pedicure is a great way to keep your toe-nails and feet clean and leave your skin soft and healthy. The best part is that you don't need to go to the spa to indulge.

## *How to do it at home*

1. Remove any existing nail polish.
2. Soak your feet in warm water for 10 minutes using a sea-salt soak. You can use this time to lower the lights and listen to soothing music, for extra pampering.
3. Use a foot file – after soaking, gently scrub all the dead skin from your feet until they are smooth.
4. File your toenails (straight across, rather than curved, for better toenail health!).
5. Buff your nails to increase the blood circulation to the nail bed and give them a smoother surface for the polish to adhere to.
6. Remove dead skin from the cuticles: use a small cuticle-pushing stick and cuticle serum to remove any dead skin; be gentle. You can

also use a cotton bud to push the cuticles; it's softer and a good alternative for sensitive skin.
7. Moisturize your feet and give yourself a loving foot massage at the same time.
8. Paint your nails (this is the fun part), and don't forget the top coat!

*Voilà* – tip-top toes for days!

# Make a Scrapbook

Let's take a trip down memory lane. If you have a bit of spare time, an empty notebook, and some glue or tape, you can enjoy the often-forgotten visceral process of sourcing, selecting and positioning photos, tickets and trinkets into a scrapbook.

Scrapbooking is all about documenting and preserving memories. Have you ever looked at old family pictures and wondered, *Who is that?* or *When was that?* This is your chance to put all your photos in a safe place and write down the names and places you can remember for your future self or descendants.

Also, if you were the kind of person that saved old flyers from your first school party, teenage love letters, beer mats, a birthday card from a special person, a magazine poster or newspaper cut-outs, and they are getting dusty in a box somewhere, you must have kept them for a reason so now is the time to give them some new-found appreciation by adding them in too.

Think how exciting it will be to flick through your scrapbook in another twenty years from now!

# Write a Freak-Out List

Often when we are freaking out we have trouble breaking down the problem (or perceived problem) into easily digestible chunks. Instead we become overwhelmed and the issue feels bigger and scarier than it really is. If this is how you feel right now and something seems too much to bear, here is one way of taking back control of your feelings: write a freak-out list using the three columns below. We've included some examples of what it might look like.

| Name the feeling | Why are you feeling this way? (Be as specific as possible.) | What can you realistically do to solve it? |
|---|---|---|
| Worry | My friend hasn't texted me after a small disagreement. | I could send a short, but kind olive branch and respect the response. |

| Sadness/ grief/ jealousy | My ex is with someone else and I still have feelings for them. | Ask myself: do I see there ever being a healthy reconciliation? If yes, maybe tell them how I feel. If no, leave them to get on with their life. Plenty of other fish in the sea. |
| --- | --- | --- |
| Fear | I am dangerously close to my overdraft this month and there are many upcoming social events I feel obliged to attend. | I could cut down on some non-essential items, like the takeaway coffees and lunches, and politely decline 50 per cent of the social events. People will understand and I am not obliged to stress myself out. |

By laying out your emotions, and your options, you can eradicate the feeling of overwhelm and take back control, which will ultimately make you happier and more confident.

Good luck – you've got this: all of it!

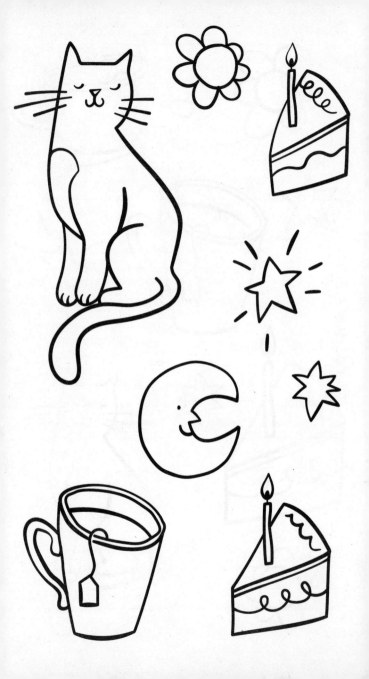

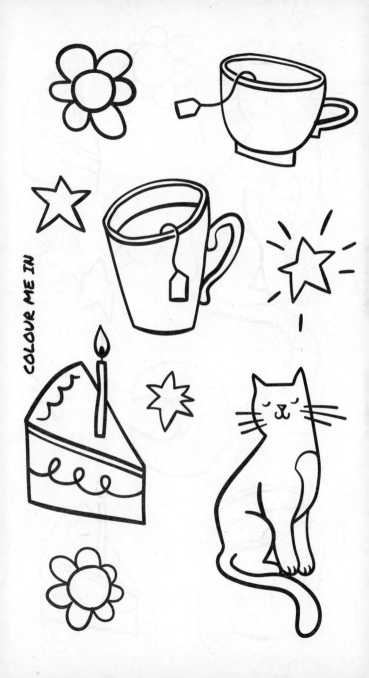

COLOUR ME IN

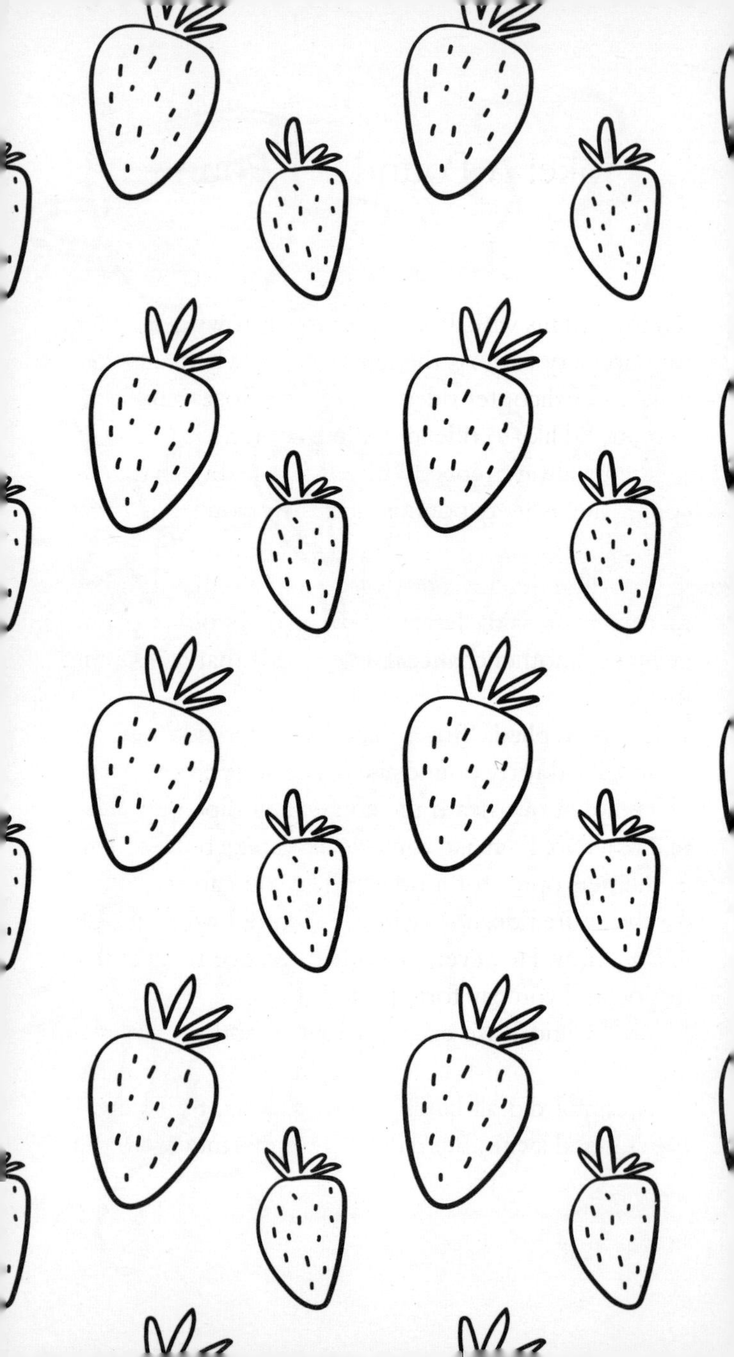

# Joke: A Pound is a Pound

Jeremy and his wife, Rose, went to the town's summer funfair every year. At the fair were big wheels, candy-floss and helicopter rides. Every year Rose would say, 'Jeremy, I'd like to ride in that helicopter.'

Jeremy always replied, 'I know, Rose, but that helicopter ride is forty pounds, and forty pounds is forty pounds.'

One year Jeremy and Rose went to the summer funfair. Rose said, 'Jeremy, I'm 79 years old. I might never get another chance if I don't ride that helicopter this year.'

Jeremy replied, 'Rose, that helicopter ride is forty pounds, and forty pounds is forty pounds.'

The pilot overheard the couple and piped up, 'Listen, you two, I'll make you a deal. I'll take both of you in the helicopter for a ride, and if you can stay quiet for the entire ride, not saying one word, I won't charge you a penny. However, just one utterance from either of you and you pay forty pounds.'

Jeremy and Rose excitedly agreed and set off into the sky.

The pilot did all kinds of fancy tricks, turns, manoeuvres and swirls, but didn't hear a murmur from the couple. Stunned, he tried his madcap antics over and over, but still not a word.

Eventually they landed, and the pilot turned to Rose. 'Blimey, I did everything I could to get you to shout out, but you didn't. I'm impressed!'

Rose said, 'Well, to be honest, I almost said something when Jeremy fell out, but you know, forty pounds is forty pounds.'

# Build Some Muscle

The whole world is a stage (or a gym, in this case) and building muscle is one of the most important aspects of long-term health and longevity. It is also a sure-fire way to get the blood pumping and to give you a boost when you feel a bit low and lethargic. The best thing is that you don't have to be a gym buff or own any equipment! Here are simple ways to build muscle using household items, while doing your daily activities:

- Grab two cans of beans from the cupboard and hold them out in front of you while the kettle boils.
- Pick up the milk from the fridge and curl your arm towards you five times. Swap arms, do the same and then pour the milk into your tea or coffee.
- Grab two cartons of juice or milk and hold them out at your sides in a wing shape for 45 seconds.

All right, calm down there, Popeye!

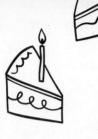

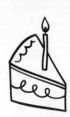
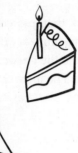

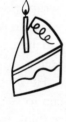
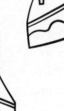

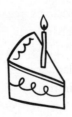
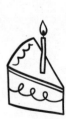
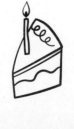

# Work This One Out . . .

Riddles are statements or questions that present the reader with a challenge. They are stimulating, as we must use critical-thinking skills to determine the answer. Try this one out and see how you like it. The answer is on the next page – try not to peek.

## Question

An agent was in Canada to gather intelligence on the best locations for future maple-syrup processing plants. The operations manager of the largest Canadian manufacturer was presented to him. But the manager was wary, so he asked the agent a question, to see whether he could be trusted. He then asked, 'What would you be absolutely certain to discover in the heart of Toronto?' The spy had to think quickly to come up with an explanation for the manager, but he did. What did he say in response?

## *Answer*

'o' – it's the middle letter in 'Toronto'.

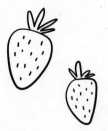

# Watch a Concert

Many people love to go to concerts to feel the rush and energy of the audience, the pulsing music and the joy of seeing the world's top musicians do their thing. However, if you can't get to one (or don't like crowds), there are many great concerts to watch or stream online, which are sure to make you feel like you are there.

Here are some recommendations for the best-recorded shows that you can watch or stream:

- Lizzo at Glastonbury (2019)
- Fleetwood Mac: *The Dance* (1997)
- Bruce Springsteen: *Western Stars* (2019)
- Queen's performance at Live Aid (1985)
- Michael Jackson (Bucharest Live Tour 1992)

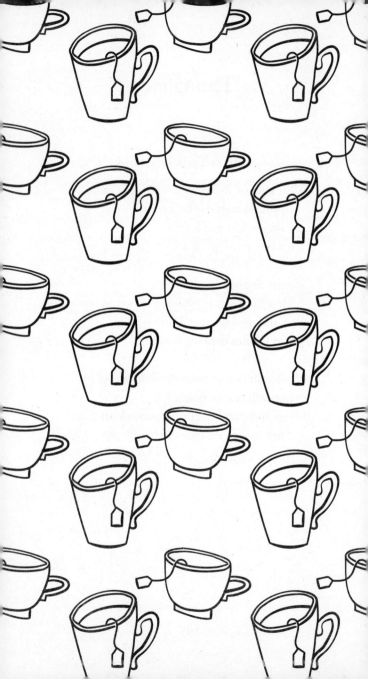

# 'Thoughts'

Myra Viola Wilds

What kind of thoughts now, do you carry
   In your travels day by day
Are they bright and lofty visions,
   Or neglected, gone astray?

Matters not how great in fancy,
   Or what deeds of skill you've wrought;
Man, though high may be his station,
   Is no better than his thoughts.

Catch your thoughts and hold them tightly,
   Let each one an honor be;
Purge them, scourge them, burnish brightly,
   Then in love set each one free.

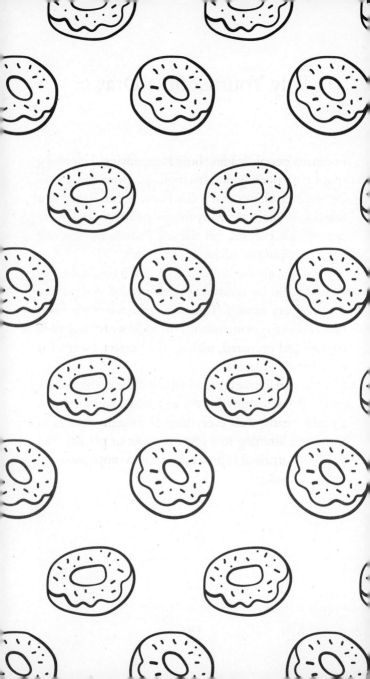

# Tidy Your Cutlery Drawer

For many people leading busy lives, tidying their living space is frequently an afterthought. However, growing research shows that a tidy home is conducive to a tidy mind. There are many things in this world that are out of our control, yet we *can* choose to tidy our homes, helping to unclutter our minds.

Although almost nobody does this, it is said that we should begin by scrubbing the inside of our cutlery drawer every month. This is because we often open that drawer to get utensils for the food we have already cooked and prepared, making it a perfect cavern for crumbs and grease.

This is an ideal excuse to take out the cutlery, shine up the forks, spoons, knives and so on, and put them all back neatly, with everything in its right place. Do this while listening to a great podcast or playlist, and you'll be surprised at how calm and accomplished you feel as a result.

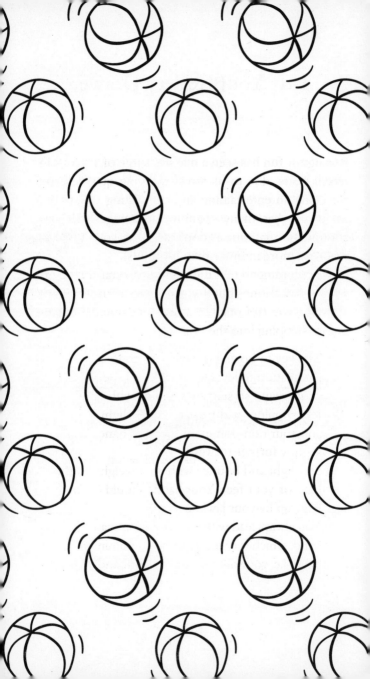

# Boxing

Boxing for fun has seen a massive surge of interest in recent years, due to its stress-relieving qualities and for being an entertaining and stimulating way to get fit. It also has many cognitive advantages, because coordination is critical (don't worry if you're bad at this – it's more intuitive than it sounds).

We recommend that the best way to start boxing is with a professional, but if you want to learn the basics at home, you can practise a few fundamental moves before stepping into the ring:

- The key to boxing is having a strong foundation to leverage power and speed from your weight so start by standing with your feet shoulder-width apart, knees slightly bent and your non-dominant foot and hand slightly further forward.
- Stay light and bouncy with your weight on the balls of your feet. Your hands should be in fists, up by your jawline.
- You always lead with your non-dominant hand, which is called 1, and your dominant hand, i.e. your right if you're right-handed, is 2.

- Try a quick sequence of jabbing your fist out in front of you (into the air – don't hit anything). Start in the boxing stance and jab, 1, 2, 1, bringing your hands back to your cheeks after each jab. Practise that sequence for a while, staying light on your toes, then you can try the same sequence with hooks and uppercuts.
- To do a hook: Bring your weight through your lead leg into your lead arm and swing that elbow out squarely behind your lead fist, so that your punch lands with your lead arm bent at the elbow and your closed fist and knuckles pointing down.
- To do an uppercut: Dip your head to the outside of your lead foot, lean in slightly, twist your hips, and spin your body upwards while delivering the lead uppercut. Your head dip is crucial for feinting and slipping a blow.
- Always snap your hand back to the starting position as quickly as possible after every punch to protect your face and head as if you were really in the ring.
- Imagine an opponent if you like (that can make this a very cathartic exercise!) but remember not to hit anything solid until you are taught properly.
- Go ahead and let your feelings roll with the punches!

# Mulled Wine

Mulled wine's popularity in Britain began in Victorian England, when it was regarded as a refined Christmas drink, and it has since been a favourite during the festive season. Delicious, comforting and perfect for warming up with on a gloomy winter day, mulled wine is, thankfully, here to stay.

Serves 6
Prep time – 10 mins

- 1 bottle light or medium-bodied red wine
- ¼ cup bourbon or brandy (optional)
- ¼ cup demerara sugar
- 2 cinnamon sticks
- 2 star anise
- 4 whole cloves
- 2 oranges, sliced

1. In a saucepan, over a medium heat, add all the ingredients and heat until almost boiling.
2. Reduce the heat to a simmer and continue to heat for 5–10 minutes, until it tastes sweet.
3. Strain into mugs so you don't drink any bits, and enjoy!

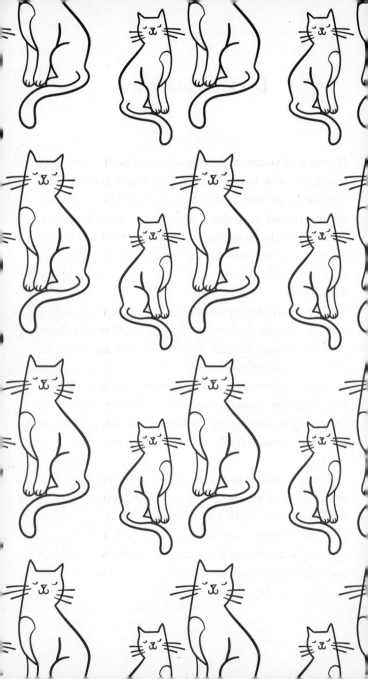

# Boost Your Ego

If you find yourself feeling low, maybe things aren't going the way you'd hoped, you aren't feeling very confident, or just a bit stuck, the likelihood is that those around you don't see things the same way. Sometimes the best way to remind ourselves of our worth is to take a loved one's word for it. After all, they probably know you better than you know yourself.

So, if you're fed up with listening to your own inner critic and in need of an ego boost, reach out to three of your closest friends and family and ask them to describe you in three words. Whether you can speak to them in person, over the phone, or simply in a text, start by showing your vulnerability, by telling them you're struggling to believe in yourself right now and could really do with hearing how they see you.

There is no doubt that your loved ones will jump at the chance to reassure you and that their responses will give you a warm hug of appreciation and love – and maybe even a real-life hug! Not only that, but by opening yourself up for a candid interaction like this you might get more than just an ego boost and deepen your relationships in the long term.

If you're worried about sounding egotistical, think about how you'd feel if your roles were reversed. We are conditioned to find helping others rewarding, so don't worry – open yourself up to love, and return the favour whenever someone else is in need.